D0456171

Health and Community Design

Health
AND
Community Design

THE IMPACT OF THE BUILT ENVIRONMENT ON PHYSICAL ACTIVITY

Lawrence D. Frank
Peter O. Engelke
Thomas L. Schmid

Island Press   WASHINGTON | COVELO | LONDON

Copyright © 2003 Lawrence D. Frank and Peter O. Engelke

All rights reserved under International and Pan-American
Copyright Conventions. No part of this book may be reproduced in
any form or by any means without permission in writing from the
publisher: Island Press, 1718 Connecticut Ave., NW, Suite 300,
Washington, DC 20009

Island Press is a trademark of The Center for Resource Economics.

Library of Congress Cataloging-in-Publication Data

Frank, Lawrence.
Health and community design : the impact of the built environment on
physical activity / Lawrence Frank, Peter Engelke, Thomas Schmid.
p.   cm.
Includes bibliographical references and index.
ISBN 1-55963-917-2 (pbk. : alk. paper)
1. Urban health. 2. Transportation—Health aspects.
3. City planning—Health aspects. 4. Health behavior.
I. Engelke, Peter. II. Schmid, Thomas. III. Title.
RA566.7.F736 2003   362.1'042—dc21
2003000999

British Cataloguing-in-Publication Data available

The contents of this book reflect the views of the authors, who are responsible
for the facts and accuracy of the findings presented herein. The contents do not
necessarily reflect the official views or policies of the Centers for
Disease Control and Prevention, the Georgia Institute of Technology,
and the University of British Columbia.

No copyright claim is made in the work of
Thomas L. Schmid, employee of the federal government.

Printed on recycled, acid-free paper ✪

Manufactured in the United States of America
09 08 07 06 05 04 03   10 9 8 7 6 5 4 3 2 1

CONTENTS

LIST OF FIGURES

LIST OF PHOTOGRAPHS

LIST OF TABLES

The idea for a book on the relationships between community design and public health arose out of the authors' research on the relationships between the built environment, travel choice, and air quality in Seattle, Washington and Atlanta, Georgia. The extension of this research into physical activity and public health was spawned by a grant provided by the Centers for Disease Control and Prevention (CDC) to Lawrence Frank and Peter Engelke at Georgia Tech in 1998, the purpose of which was to review the literature on public health on the one hand and transportation, urban design, and city planning on the other. In so doing, it was hoped that this research would help to clarify the commonalities between these seemingly disparate fields and assist in the development of a comprehensive research agenda. This grant led the CDC to participate in a larger research program called SMARTRAQ (Strategies for Metropolitan Atlanta's Regional Transportation and Air Quality), which is a $4.6 million regional study focused on transportation, land use, air quality, and public health. The incorporation of a health-based research agenda into SMARTRAQ is a unique feature of this regional transportation and land use study and reflects the understanding possessed by the program's funding agencies of the health effects of growth and development in the Atlanta region. The authors are, therefore, extremely appreciative of the support provided by the study's primary sponsoring agencies, the Georgia Department of Transportation and the Georgia Regional Transportation Authority. To this end, we would like to thank the principals within these agencies who have been instrumental in putting together a health-oriented research program for the Atlanta region, in particular George Boulineau and Charles Fleming. Additionally, the authors would like to thank the Turner Foundation for providing the grants that allowed us to spend time conducting background research on related topics and to write this manuscript. Particular thanks in this context go to Douglas Stewart.

The CDC has a long-standing interest in policy and environmental approaches to the prevention and control of disease and associated conditions. Our interest in the relationships between community design and health-enhancing behaviors such as physical activity came to a clear focus as a result of an event sponsored by the CDC in 1998 in Atlanta, Georgia, which included a panel discussion on policy and environmental actions to promote physical activity. This panel included "non-traditional" public health partners as well as representatives from the fields of transportation, community design, criminology, environmental protection, and architecture. The research agenda that emerged as a result of this meeting has guided the efforts of the CDC's Division of Nutrition and Physical Activity, Active Community Environments (ACEs) workgroup. This book is one of the first tangible products of these efforts. It and the ACEs research portfolio could not have been developed without the intellectual, administrative, and financial support of William Dietz and David Buchner. This is also true of Michael Pratt, who along with Richard Killingsworth and Thomas Schmid are founding members of the ACEs workgroup.

An undertaking such as this would not have been possible were it not for the hard work and valuable contributions of numerous individuals. The staff at Island Press worked diligently to move this book from rough draft to finished product. Particular thanks need to be given to our editor at Island Press, Heather Boyer. Heather's insight and suggestions greatly improved the style and content of our manuscript, while her patience with the inevitable delays involved in producing the finished manuscript was much appreciated.

We would like to recognize the contributions made by Christopher Leerssen of the SMARTRAQ program at Georgia Tech. His work made the images contained in this book possible. This is not an insignificant task—as the reader will see, this book contains a large number of graphics. Each had to be created from scratch, adapted from another source, or simply improved in terms of content or style. The high quality of the images is the direct result of Christopher's considerable abilities.

We are also appreciative of the insights and observations of many people who influenced the ideas and research that form the basis for this book. These individuals provided intellectual assistance during the course of numerous conversations and, thus, influenced our musings on the subjects contained in this book in one way or another. These individuals include Howard Frumkin, Gayle Nelson, James Sallis, Brian Saelens, Chris Leinberger, Gregg Logan, Richard Jackson, Jim Chapman, Jim Durrett, Anne Vernez-Moudon, Walter Brown, Jonathan Levine, Jack Feldman, and John Pucher. Particular thanks go to Jonathan Levine, whose review of the manuscript yielded many valuable suggestions.

During the course of our background research, we have relied on numerous sources, including academic journal articles, books, reports issued by government agencies and nonprofit organizations, and excerpts from the speeches and journals of historical figures. As are all scholars, we are deeply indebted to the organizations that published these materials and to the individuals who created them. We are solely responsible for any errors, omissions, misinterpretations, or misrepresentations of their work.

CHAPTER ONE

Introduction

We ought to plan the ideal of our city with an eye to four considerations.
The first, as being the most indispensable, is health.

ARISTOTLE,
Politics (ca. 350 B.C.)

Community design influences human behavior. The ways that cities, sub-urbs, and towns are designed and built impact the people who work, live, and play in them. The placement, layout, and design of transportation systems, of office complexes, of parks, and of the countless physical elements that make up communities result in real places that have real significance in terms of how we spend our time and what activities we engage in. Where people live, where they work, how they get around, how much pollution they produce, what kinds of environmental hazards they face, and what kinds of amenities they enjoy are a direct product of how communities are designed. This book is about how our communities influence one important type of behavior, physical activity, and the health outcomes that are associated with it.

Unfortunately, the great majority of Americans do not get enough physical activity to maintain their health over the long run. Physical inactivity is an enormous health problem in this country, contributing to, among other things, premature death, chronic disease, osteoporosis, poor mental health, and obesity. The environments in which most people spend their time—the modern American city and the suburbs and exurbs that have been the dominant form of development in this country for over a half century—are an important contributor to this problem. The cities and suburbs that we inhabit are not now, and have not been for a long time, places that encourage some critically important forms of physical activity. In short, our physical environment inhibits many forms of activity, such as walking, and has become a significant barrier to more active lifestyles.

A century ago, American cities were highly walkable places. They were compact. Commercial, retail, and even industrial operations existed in close proximity to housing, allowing people to walk to work or school or the store. Out of necessity, buildings and streets were designed to the human scale. Streetcar and trolley systems provided a major form of transportation for millions of passengers every day, in every major city in the nation, which meant that people had the means to make longer journeys without the use of a car. When combined, all of this produced environments in which someone could satisfy their basic daily needs within a comfortable walking distance of their home or within a distance reachable through a combination of walking and trolley riding.

Unfortunately, the burgeoning cities of the industrial era also brought with them a host of serious problems. They were dirty and polluted. They were crowded. Most importantly, they produced health problems for their inhabitants. The worst of these were the communicable disease epidemics—typhus, yellow fever, and all manner of other infectious diseases—that swept through them with frightening regularity. The very conditions that made the industrial city a highly walkable place, including its concentration of people, its mixing of uses, and its high density of buildings, came to be blamed—not quite accurately, as research eventually showed—for creating the conditions in which epidemics could occur. So during the nineteenth and early twentieth centuries, critics tore away at the intellectual foundation of the compact industrial city. They sought to replace it with a new paradigm, a new way of thinking about how to build cities. In the old city's place they created the modern decentralized city, where housing was separated from workplaces and buildings placed far apart from one another, separated by expanses of grass and trees. America's new cities of big lawns and big distances would, they hoped and expected, produce more healthy living. What resulted was the city that we are so familiar with today—dominated by suburbs, spread out, with different uses separated one from another and almost everything reliant on automobile travel. This mass suburbanization also led directly to a decline, in terms of population, wealth, and public investment in the older, established central parts of most cities, resulting in the widespread abandonment of the fabric of the old walkable city.

Widespread criticism of this development model has appeared only during the last couple of decades. Much of it is a reaction to the omnipresent automobile congestion that is the hallmark of the decentralized city. Some of it is centered on the monstrous-yet-monotonous ugliness of the endless strip malls and parking lots that have proliferated from one end of the country to the other. Many people are concerned about the environmental consequences of the modern city. These concerns focus on the enormous amount of land consumed, the air quality problems produced by all of the cars needed to keep these cities running, the vast quantities of municipal water that is required to irrigate the lawns of the new suburban landscapes, or the rainwater that is wasted as polluted runoff from parking lots and streets. An even more recent source of criticism is from the field of public health, which is beginning to explore potentially uncomfortable linkages between the decentralized city and different indicators of health.

Physical Activity, Past and Present

In the old cities, getting enough physical activity during one's day wasn't an issue because it was as much a part of life as eating or sleeping. Today, physical activity has been engineered out of most aspects of life. Work is no longer physically demanding for most people and daily living patterns, from mowing the grass to cooking dinner to washing clothes, require significantly less manual effort than they once did. The modern city has changed all of this, creating environments in which it is less and less common to work physical activity into the everyday patterns of life. The dominant forms of community design have contributed to this decline by making walking and cycling for transportation difficult if not impossible. Many of the reasons why are clear to even the casual observer. Long distances between places mean that most people cannot walk or bicycle from one place to another. The streets and roads that connect these far-flung places are designed for cars, often making them unsafe and extremely unattractive for pedestrians and bicyclists. To make matters worse, most developers and retailers have long given up on the profitability of designing places that are visually attractive to people who might want to walk from place to place, favoring instead designs that attract motorists. As a result, being physically active now requires planning for activities such as running, biking, aerobics, or weight lifting that can be done during leisure time.

Coincidentally, during the post–World War II period, public health research came to focus more and more on recreational and vigorous physical activity as the way to improve public health. For years, health experts recommended that each individual get at least twenty minutes of high-intensity exercise each day. The basic idea was that anything less would result in little or no improvement in long-term health. And, judging by the attention paid to such forms of exercise in the popular media, it would seem that vigorous physical activity has been a runaway success. Specialty magazines devoted to participatory sports and exercise programs ranging from running to weight lifting to climbing jam the racks at newsstands. An array of televised sports occupies much of the country's attention on weekends, bringing basketball, football, hockey, baseball, and a slew of other offerings into millions of homes. Advertisers in the print and electronic media perpetually barrage the country with images of the perfectly fit human figure, both male and female.

Yet this picture of a fit and healthy society is enormously misleading. The fact is that most Americans don't get enough physical activity to meet the health recommendations set by public health agencies. Despite the omnipresence of televised sports, the billions of dollars in exercise equipment and apparel sold every year, the millions of words published on fitness and exercise regimens, and the endless rhetoric springing from athletic shoe and apparel companies' advertising campaigns, only about five percent of the population—*one person in twenty*—gets enough physical activity through vigorous exercise to satisfy public health standards (CDC 2001b). Even worse, some studies have found that as much as 40 percent of the population is sedentary (being completely inactive) (Schoenborn and Barnes 2002); they report that they get no physical activity at all during their leisure hours. For all of the promotion and attention paid to sports- and gym-based exercise as the way to get people physically fit, the great majority of the population has not succeeded in becoming physically active through these means. While millions of people do get a great deal of health benefit as well as personal satisfaction from sports, from training for endurance and strength events, and from going to the gym for a workout, many more find that they don't have the will or the ability or the time or the resources to do any of these things.

These are some of the reasons why, beginning in the 1980s and continuing into the 1990s, public health agencies and researchers began to take a serious look at more moderate types of physical activity such as walking and bicycling. Mounting evidence from epidemiological studies began to reveal that moderate forms of physical activity could provide both short- and long-term health benefits, contributing to a reduction in the risk of premature mortality, chronic disease, and a host of other maladies. Moreover, public health researchers began to believe that a focus on more moderate forms of physical activity might enable a broader cross-section of the population to become physically active. Because moderate physical activity is lower in intensity, it is easier for a person who is sedentary to begin and to maintain their participation over the long term. Moderate physical activity can be purposive, meaning that it can be integrated into daily living habits, and as a result it should be more attractive to people who don't have the necessary free time to work out at a gym or go mountain biking in the woods.

What is old, then, is new: public health agencies now endorse those forms of moderate physical activity such as walking and bicycling that used to be very commonplace in American cities and towns. Public health officials recommend that people accumulate at least thirty minutes of moderate activity on most, preferably all days of the week. Adding any additional amount of moderate activity is good; in fact, while public health agencies recommend trying to get at least thirty minutes per day, there is a belief that even ten or twenty additional minutes per day might generate some benefits. Vigorous physical activity is still considered to be an important means of staying healthy, but public health experts now believe that adding a half hour or more of moderate physical activity per day on most days of the week is enough to generate long-term health benefits.

This consensus opinion carries enormous significance for addressing the problem of physical inactivity. It suggests—perhaps demands—that public health agencies not limit themselves to programs that rely solely on motivating individuals to take up vigorous exercise. Rather, the door has been opened for an examination of the environmental influences of moderate physical activity. If one needs a half hour or more of moderate physical activity per day, accumulated in numerous short bouts, it might be wise to focus on creating environments that allow these types of activities to occur as a matter of course, as incidental to doing other things. For many people, perhaps even the majority of the population, such an approach may be the only realistic way to increase physical activity (incidentally, increasing physical activity in this way may also be a way to reduce automobile use and lessen its attendant problems, such as air pollution and congestion). For different segments of the population who are disadvantaged—many elderly and physically handicapped people, for instance—vigorous activities may be out of the question completely. For physically capable people in the prime of life, other obstacles such as a lack of time may severely constrict their ability to work out on a regular basis. For the significant percentage of the population that is sedentary, the benefits of adding a half hour of moderate physical activity each day is enormous: physical activity follows a dose-response curve, wherein the marginal benefits to increased exercise accrue the most to those who are the least active to begin with (see chapter 3).

Community Design, Physical Activity, and Health: A Conceptual Model

Figure 1-1 provides a simple model of the relationships between physical activity, health, and the environments in which people live and work. This is the basic conceptual model for the chapters to follow. Causality flows, roughly, from the built environment (the communities in which we live and environments in which we work) through physical activity patterns to public health outcomes. Physical activity is at the literal as well as conceptual center of the model, providing the linkage between the real, built environment and the health outcomes that are of such concern to public health officials.

The built environment denotes the form and character of communities. It is made up of the countless specific places—homes, streets, offices, parking lots, shopping malls, restaurants, parks, movie theaters—that constitute a city or town or suburb. Our model utilizes three broad categories—transportation systems, land use patterns, and urban design characteristics—to provide coherence to the built environment. Transportation systems connect places to each other, determining how feasible it is to use different types of transportation, including walking and bicycling, to get from one place to another. Local transportation systems are impacted by major investments in highways, airports, and other infrastructure decisions

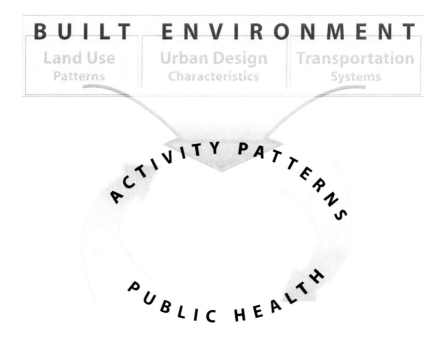

FIGURE 1-1. Model of linkages between the built environment, physical activity, and public health

made by regional and state officials. Land use patterns consist of the arrangement of residences, offices, restaurants, grocery stores, and other places within the built environment. The arrangement of these activities, or land uses, determine how close different places such as housing, work, and entertainment are to one another, thereby making journeys on foot or by bicycle practical or impractical. They also shape physical activity patterns through the distribution of open space and recreational facilities where sports and other activities can take place. Finally, urban design characteristics influence how people perceive the built environment. Design plays a large role in determining whether an environment is perceived as hostile or friendly, attractive or ugly, and vibrant or dull. Urban design denotes small-scale features of the built environment that impact how people feel about being in specific places.

The conceptual model provided in figure 1-1 illustrates the interactive nature between one's health and the environment in which one lives, works, and engages in other activities. The arrows that run in both directions between physical activity and health denote how physical activity is both a cause and an effect. The arrow extending from public health to physical activity reflects the likelihood that some health outcomes, such as high levels of obesity or chronic disease in the population, may make it harder for some people to engage in physical activity. Basically, the poorer the health of the population, the more difficult it becomes to increase physical activity levels. However, our central focus is on how the built environment influences physical activity levels.

This leads to a second observation on causality in the model: physical activity is only one contributor, albeit a very important one, to health outcomes. There are, of course, many other reasons why people suffer from ill health. To take one example, during the 1990s and into the new century, the high rates of obesity in the United States became the focus of much research within public health circles as well as a favorite subject of the press. Obesity has multiple causes, ranging from genetics to poor diet to environmental factors and personal behavior. While one's genetics are an important determinant of obesity, diet and physical activity are things that can be controlled. The built environment impacts both of these behaviors. (While we focus on physical activity in this book, the location of quality food outlets versus fast food venues is another way that the built environment impacts our health; in poorer parts of cities, for example, there tend to be fewer food establishments—restaurants and grocery stores—serving healthy foods.) As tempting as it is to point to the built environment as a main cause of problems such as obesity, it is not acceptable to draw a straight line between the two and imply that only environmental improvement will solve the problem; clearly there are other determinants of obesity.

Nonetheless, the intent of this book is to argue that most of the communities where Americans live are important contributors to current public health problems. Simultaneously, they can also be the source of important solutions to these problems. Communities can be designed to make physical activity in them possible and even desirable. Environments that encourage moderate physical activity may also have features that make them more livable in other ways, by improving one's quality of life—they may generate more social interaction, foster less dependence on the automobile, be safer for their inhabitants, and give people more choices with respect to how they get around and spend their time. In these pages we do not seek to condemn any particular form of community design. Rather, a central goal is to develop a better understanding of the ways in which the features of the built environment serve to encourage or discourage health-promoting behaviors, two of which are walking and bicycling. Public policies that influence how to build communities—which zoning and building codes to adopt, which transportation systems to build, and so on—can best be understood and assessed once the health benefits and costs of such choices are included in the calculus.

The Plan of the Book

The rest of the book addresses in more detail the multiple themes introduced in this chapter. Chapter 2 provides background for understanding how the built environments in which Americans live and work have come to exist and emphasizes how public health considerations during the nineteenth and twentieth centuries shaped, in a critical way, thinking about how to design cities. Ironically, these considerations helped to legitimize the new decentralized cities of the mid- to late twentieth century, cities that are now contributing to the public health problems of the twenty-first century. Chapters 3 and 4 set the foundation for the arguments about the physical design of our communities and our regions that follow later in the book: they lay out the case as to why moderate types of physical activity, in particular walking and bicycling, should be a focus of public policies. Chapter 5 focuses on the divergent needs and requirements that different groups of people have with respect to physical activity and argues that some groups of people, including children, the elderly, and the poor, have difficulties negotiating the built environment and therefore possess divergent needs and requirements with respect to how the built environment is designed and built. Chapters 6 through 10 detail how the built environment influences levels of physical activity, with the primary focus on how different settings make it easier or more difficult to walk and bicycle for practical journeys. A concluding chapter focuses on the prospects for changing the built environment to make it more conducive to physical activity.

Finally, while this book utilizes information and data from many cities, the reader will note that two cities, Atlanta and Seattle, receive the greatest amount of attention. The authors of the book have been conducting research in these cities for a number of years and have, therefore, a more thorough understanding of the subtle problems and distinctions involving the built environment in these places. Yet the inclusion of examples from these cities is also not random: Atlanta and Seattle provide important case studies because of the degree of urban form contrast between them. These distinctions are drawn most clearly in chapter 10, but are also referenced intermittently throughout the book.

CHAPTER TWO

Public Health and Urban Form in America

HISTORICAL PRECEDENTS

The Decentrists hammered away at the bad old city. They were incurious about successes in great cities. They were interested only in failures. . . . The Decentrists' analyses, the architectural and housing designs which were companions and off-shoots of these analyses, the national housing and home financing legislation so directly influenced by the new vision— none of these had anything to do with understanding cities, or fostering successful large cities, nor were they expected to. They were reasons and means for jettisoning cities.

JANE JACOBS,
The Death and Life of Great American Cities (1961)

The modern American city's basic form—decentralized, dispersed, containing separated land uses and autocentric transportation networks— has its origins in deliberate attempts to remake and refashion urban America during a long period extending from roughly the middle of the nineteenth century into the middle of the twentieth. During this time a wide range of architects, planners, activists, politicians, and other professionals sought to forge orderly, safe, and efficient cities out of the chaos of the industrial era. Movements for reform originated out of the extreme conditions produced by increasing urbanization and industrialization and gained strength rapidly by the last third of the nineteenth century. The nineteenth century urban landscape was, by most accounts, extremely unpleasant: crowded, dirty, polluted, smelly, noisy, and dangerous. These public health concerns led to an ideal of the horizontal city that was characterized by decentralized settlement patterns, the separation of dissimilar land uses, and dominated by the idea that public policy ought to support and protect neighborhoods consisting of single family housing in leafy suburbs.[1] Indeed, the horizontal, decentralized city was conceptualized and sold as the archetype of the healthy city.

Admittedly, health was only one of several considerations that drove changes in thinking about the city during this period. Nonetheless it contributed, in a fundamental way, to the formation of a societal consensus about how the modern city ought to be built. In this chapter we discuss how public health considerations influenced the thought of key figures who were involved, directly and indirectly, in shaping urban form during the nineteenth and twentieth centuries. We select four different periods to highlight the importance of public health in shaping urban form: the movement for sanitation reform in the nineteenth century; the movement for tenement housing reform at the turn of the century; the establishment of zoning as a standard planning tool in the first decades of the twentieth century; and the evolution of the garden suburb in the nascent professional specialization of city planning—from the Garden City of Ebenezer Howard in the 1890s through the glorification of this ideal in the minds of America's leading planners in the 1920s and 1930s.

Physician Reformers: Sanitation and the Industrial City in the Nineteenth Century

During the period stretching from about 1820 through the end of the century, industrialization, trade, and migration caused sweeping changes in the size, form, and demographic composition of cities around the world, first in England and later in continental Europe and the United States. In the United States, the urban population grew from about 300,000 in 1800, to 6.2 million in 1860, and 54 million by 1920, while the percentage of the total population living in cities increased from 6 percent in 1800 to 51 percent in 1920. In-migration fueled much of the increase, of course, as the pull of the cities attracted large numbers of migrants from rural areas, but foreign immigration also accounted for a large share. During the nineteenth century, some 35 million immigrants arrived in the United States, most of whom settled in America's booming industrial cities. By 1910, 41 percent of city dwellers were first-generation immigrants (Melosi 1980). The concentration of huge populations of new migrants in the nation's burgeoning cities over the course of the nineteenth century led to some very real problems including widespread poverty and crowded, unsafe, and unsanitary housing. Many began to fear that the conditions in dense urban centers had the potential to destabilize society. Elites in the United States and Europe viewed the huge and volatile underclass that had been created by mass industrialization and mass internal and international migration as a potentially revolutionary and even violent force. The urban poor did, in fact, threaten to play such a role, through organized means such as the industrial labor movement or via sporadic and disorganized ones such as riots (Hall 1996).

Overlaid against this background were a number of troubling health considerations. By concentrating large numbers of the poor into cities and exposing them to the hardships of the early industrial era, the industrial city exacerbated centuries-old public health problems. Chief among these were epidemics of contagious diseases such as typhus, cholera, smallpox, and yellow fever. Beginning in the late eighteenth century and continuing through the nineteenth, physicians began to associate disease incidence with the particulars of urban geography (Duffy 1978). They noticed that disease often originated and spread most rapidly in the industrial city's poorest neighborhoods, as these were the areas most beset by offensive, dirty, and foul conditions (Schultz 1989). As early as the 1790s, for example, physicians had associated the outbreak of a typhus epidemic in Manchester, England, one of the world's first industrial cities, with working conditions in that city's cotton mills (Rosen 1958). In 1837, an American physician, Dr. Benjamin McCready, assigned blame for the ill health of New York's poor to the living conditions in the city's tenements (Duffy 1968).

In noticing that disease epidemics tended to originate in the city's densest and dirtiest neighborhoods, many physicians saw evidence in support of an ancient theory of disease etiology. The theory of miasma held that "poor atmospheres" caused disease, a belief that had enjoyed prominence within medicine since classical antiquity. According to this line of reasoning, unsanitary environments produced noxious gases that, when inhaled, were believed to be the method by which a person contracted a disease (Rosen 1958).

As a result, interest in sanitation reform began in earnest from the middle of the nineteenth century on both sides of the Atlantic. Sanitation reformers attacked unhealthy living conditions within the city, especially for the poor, and were central to the creation, by mid-century in the United States, of many basic public health institutions, including state boards of health and public health associations for medical professionals. Perhaps the most famous and important development in this regard occurred in 1864 with the creation of the Council of Hygiene and Public Health in New York, whose membership included many of that city's most prominent physicians, including John Griscom, Elisha Harris, Joseph Smith, and Stephen Smith. The Council, tasked with determining the causes of epidemic diseases within the city, issued a report the following year showing that the highest rates of illness and mortality were found in those parts of the city that were the dirtiest, the most crowded, and where the poorest sanitary infrastructure was located. In concluding that the conditions found in these areas caused disease, the report called for the elimination of the sources of noxious gases, such as dirty streets and overflowing sewers (Duffy 1968). The Council's report strongly influenced the passage of the landmark New York Metropolitan Health Bill of 1866, which created a Board of Health empowered with overseeing sanitation in the city. For the first time in the city's history, this legislation established a professional health administration that had the statutory guidance, expertise, and resources necessary to combat sanitation problems. This legislation became the basis for similar efforts nationwide (Brieger 1978; Rosen 1958).

Critically, the sanitation reform movement was not confined to the medical community. It had important linkages to architecture and landscape architecture, finding its most significant voice in the work of Frederick Law Olmsted. Olmsted is best known as the designer of New York's Central Park, but his significance for the American city extends well beyond Central Park and its legacy. He planned and designed several suburbs, led the nascent urban parks movement, and published widely, both as a journalist and as a landscape architect. During the Civil War, Olmsted was the secretary of the U.S. Sanitary Commission, which was charged with gathering and disseminating medical advice to physicians in field hospitals. Olmsted was certainly exposed, at the latest by the time of his appointment as the secretary of the commission, to the theory of miasma. Members of the commission issued reports on field sanitation that upheld the basic premises of the miasmatic position. One report, for example, stated that camps should be located away from marshes and other "malarious areas." Olmsted's essays written after the war clearly show that miasmatic theory informed his work on questions of urban design, in particular the ways that dense cities created the foul air he believed caused illness. In a remarkable essay written in 1868 with his long-time business partner Calvert Vaux, Olmsted linked poor health and disease to the city, and in particular to the failure of urban designers to create the conditions by which "sickening" and "deadly" gases could be eliminated. Improvements in the health of urban dwellers, he wrote, would result from the "abandonment of the old-fashioned compact way of building towns, and the gradual adoption of a custom of laying them out with much larger spaces open to the sun-light and fresh air." Olmsted blamed narrow streets and over-crowding in particular for creating the environmental conditions in which disease could flourish. Evidence for this proposition was "found in the fact that differing proportions between the dying and the living, the sick and the well, which are found to exist between towns where most of the people still live on narrow streets . . . and between parts of the same town which are most crowded and those which are more open" (Sutton 1971, 36–7).[2]

Olmsted attacked those aspects of urban design that led to overcrowding, poor drainage, and the lack of sanitation. He argued that trees and other plants had a sanitizing effect on their immediate environment (Fein 1967; Szczygiel and Hewitt 2000).[3] Open spaces were a necessary part of the healthy urban environment because they both helped to reduce the density of struc-tures over a given area and because they created spaces within the confines of the city for trees and plants. Olmsted doubted whether traditional cities, with their high densities and intense concentration of structures, could ever be locales for healthy living. In his view, "the two great natural agents of disin-fection, sunshine and foliage" could not be introduced in sufficient quantities in such places because they "cannot act largely and freely throughout the streets, and on each side of every house" (Fein 1967).[4] Parks provided foliage, opened up the city to light, and provided citizens with a much-needed escape from the "cramped, confined and controlling circumstances of the streets of the town." Wide boulevards performed many of the same functions. Finally, suburbs, connected to the city by these boulevards, had the potential to offer urban amenities "with the special charms and substantial advantages of rural conditions of life" (Fein 1967; Sutton 1971).[5]

Olmsted's contributions to the evolution of urban form went well beyond that of other sanitation reformers. As a landscape architect, he specifically linked health problems to the basic design attributes of urban spaces. If the crowded city, with its manufacturing, its poor sewage systems, its narrow streets, and its masses of urban poor, produced the conditions in which disease originated and spread, in Olmsted's view the solution was the redesign of the city according to a different model. In many respects his vision presaged the twentieth-century American city. His model had at its center the introduction of more open spaces into the city, in the form of parks, wider streets, and lot and building redesign. More importantly, Olmsted saw the prototype suburb as a design solution for the urban health problem. Olmsted contributed to the view that the low-density city, consisting of wide boulevards and parks and ringed by satellite suburbs, was the ideal urban form.

Health and Morality: Housing Reform and Progressives, 1900–1914

Reformers of the Progressive era launched a new round of attacks on the social, political, and economic conditions of the late nineteenth and early twentieth centuries. Like the physician reformers from earlier in the nineteenth century, Progressive reformers also attached great importance to the unfortunate coincidence of poverty, unsanitary housing, and overcrowding in the nation's largest cities. As had their earlier counterparts, these reformers believed that the conditions of the poor in the industrial city led to the physical and moral degradation of America's large underclass, in particular the country's enormous immigrant population.

However, by the time the Progressive housing reform movement began in earnest around the turn of the century, the medical basis that supported the case for reform along public health lines had changed considerably. During the last quarter of the nineteenth century, medical researchers had definitively established that the worst epidemic diseases, including cholera, typhoid, malaria, and tuberculosis, were caused not by poor atmospheres but by bacteria spread through contagious infection. The bacteriological breakthroughs of this period—basically the discovery of germs in the laboratory—revived the theory of contagion, which held that disease infection was transmitted from person to person by "contagia," minute agents that are transmissible. An Italian physician had first articulated this theory in the sixteenth century but it remained the minority position within the medical profession until the scientific advances of the late nineteenth century proved the truth of its basic premises (Rosen 1958).[6] Bacteriology had a profound impact on the fields of medicine and public health. Disease infection, it was now finally understood, was the result of bacterial transmission from one person to another, either through personal contact or through a medium such as a mosquito or a municipal water supply.

Earlier housing reformers had made their case for public health on the grounds that better municipal sanitation would improve health by purifying the local atmosphere. Their understanding of disease transmission led them to work for the elimination of the sources that they believed caused poor local atmospheres: dirt, filth, and noxious gases. But the bacteriological revolution had the potential to undermine the argument that linked questions of urban form to health, at least with respect to public sanitation, because it downplayed the contribution of local conditions in causing disease. Some public health officials, in fact, began shifting their health messages to themes involving personal cleanliness, even to the point of expressing frustration with the continuing popularity of the idea that poor municipal sanitation was an important cause of disease transmission (American Public Health Association 1977).[7]

However, the housing reformers of the Progressive era remained convinced that housing questions and public health problems were causally linked in American cities. They built much of their argument for reform upon tuberculosis, asserting that the tuberculosis bacteria depended upon certain environmental conditions in order to survive. At this time, physicians subscribed to the theory that sunlight and air would kill the bacteria while, conversely, dark and poorly ventilated conditions would allow them to thrive (American Public Health Association 1977; Taylor 1974).[8] These were precisely the conditions found in New York's tenements, which tended to be located in districts with high rates of tuberculosis infection. For this reason, housing reformers found that their interests in reform dovetailed nicely with those of the antituberculosis movement, which had been formed during the 1890s by physicians in Philadelphia and New York, and the work of the two groups often converged (Fairbanks 1985; Lubove 1962; Rosen 1958). The association of tuberculosis infection with urban poverty provided a public health foundation for rebuilding urban spaces. Like the arguments that had rested upon the theory of miasma, this foundation allowed reformers to argue that environmental conditions allowed disease to spread rapidly.

The most famous Progressive era housing reformer was Jacob Riis, a Danish immigrant whose influential book, *How the Other Half Lives* (1890), vividly portrayed the miserable living conditions in New York's tenements, often mere blocks from prosperous New York residences. However, while Riis and other reformers such as Mary Simkhovitch and Mary Kelley were very important, Lawrence Veiller was arguably the most critical figure in the history of the Progressive movement for housing reform. He was a tireless activist involved in nearly every question relating to housing, serving on a variety of critical boards and commissions and leaving behind a substantial body of written material. Throughout his career, Veiller would make the sunlight-and-air theme a centerpiece of his critique of the high-density urban tenement, always because he blamed the lack thereof for the spread of tuberculosis.[9] As photograph 2-1 shows, tenement buildings at the time, which collectively housed tens of thousands of mostly poor immigrants in New York, were designed in such a way that most of the apartments were dark and unventilated. Because tenement owners wished to maximize their return on investment, they sought to construct their buildings so as to occupy as much of the lot as possible, thereby containing the largest number of rentable units possible. Unfortunately, these features of the tenement's design also made it impossible for light and fresh air to penetrate into the majority of the rooms in the tenement building (Veiller 1910). Frequently, the only sources of light for many apartments were narrow "light shafts," vertical slits that ran from the ground through the ceiling of the building (photo 2-2). These shafts would not have existed at all had it not been for earlier tenement legislation requiring their use.

In a two-volume report of the New York Tenement House Commission chaired by Veiller and his colleague, Robert DeForest, published in 1903, the authors focused on "the greatest evil of the present day," the lack of light and air in these tenements. "As a result of this lack of light and air, we find that the dread disease of pulmonary tuberculosis has become practically epidemic in the city," they wrote. Referencing the testimony of a large number of physicians who had testified before the committee, they contended that "the conditions in the tenement houses were directly responsible for the tremendous extent and spread of this contagious disease," and that the first step to take was increasing the amount of light and air in the buildings (DeForest and Veiller 1903).[10]

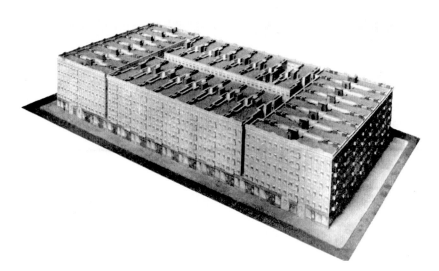

PHOTO 2-1. Manhattan's tenements were the focus of housing reform for much of the nineteenth and early twentieth centuries. Tenement designs such as this were dark, poorly ventilated, and very crowded. Source: DeForest and Veiller, 1903. Copyright Ayer Company Publishers, 1 Lower Mill Road, North Stratford, NH, 03590. Reprinted with permission.

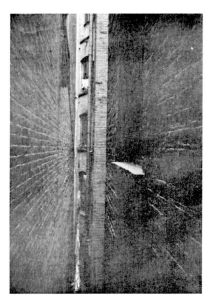

PHOTO 2-2. The only source of light and fresh air for many tenements was the "light shaft," narrow slits running from the ground through the ceiling, and can also be seen in figure 1. These were mandated by law in the nineteenth century to provide some light to interior apartments but by the late nineteenth century had become a symbol of everything that was wrong with the tenement. Source: DeForest and Veiller, 1903. Copyright Ayer Company Publishers, 1 Lower Mill Road, North Stratford, NH, 03590. Reprinted with permission.

Like many of his contemporaries, Veiller also believed that the tenement bred moral illness. In the Tenement House Commission report, Veiller had ascribed "grave moral and social dangers" to the endemic poverty and squalor of the tenements (Veiller 1903). He later wrote that the tenement "leaves its ineffaceable records on the souls, minds and bodies of men, there to be read by all to understand." A child growing up in the tenements "does not grow up to be a normal person" and "is handicapped in his school life; his earning capacity is diminished and his resisting power weakened." Of the social dangers, he stated flatly: "it is not of such material that strong nations are made. . . . Democracy was not predicated upon a country made up of tenement dwellers, nor can it so survive" (Lubove 1967).

For these reasons, Veiller wanted the housing reform debate to address the ways that architecture and urban design could contribute to improvements in all of the dimensions of health—physical, moral, and psychological. His primary solution was to attack the problem through legislation. He advocated limitations on building heights, lot depth, block sizes, and street layout, and later became interested in questions involving the zoning of the entire city. In his view, there were only two ways to guarantee that sufficient light and air would reach building inhabitants. The first was to force builders to conform to guidelines for the construction of buildings with respect to the dimensions of the lot. This required restrictions on the maximum height of buildings as well as the introduction of setback requirements to the front, rear, and side of all buildings. The result would be shorter buildings set farther apart from one another. The second way was to redesign the city block itself so as to banish certain types of lots. In particular, this meant the prohibition in tenement districts of the deep and narrow lot—lots which were 125 feet in depth but perhaps only 40 feet across, dimensions that made it difficult to introduce light and air from the sides and rear of the tenement. Veiller reasoned, very accurately, that the street plan determined the shape and dimension of the block, which then determined the possible lot sizes and dimensions. To prevent tenements from being too deep front-to-back (which had the effect of increasing the number of interior apartments), blocks needed to be redesigned so as to be wide from left to right but shallow from front to back (Veiller 1911).

Veiller tied changes in building and lot design to the tenement problem throughout his entire career. In this respect, his work was an important contributor to the idea of the ideal city that was beginning to coalesce within the field of city planning at the time of his writing. According to this ideal, good housing required the separation of buildings from each other and from the streets on which they fronted. His codes were forerunners to New York's first zoning ordinance of 1916 and became the basis for state and municipal housing codes across the United States (Lubove 1962; Toll 1969; Willis 1993). More generally, the housing reform movement of which Veiller was a part made an important contribution to the idea that high concentrations of structures and people made for unhealthy living. They helped to forge ideas that became accepted as axiomatic in the minds of subsequent generations of planners and public health officials. Housing and health came to be linked in two specific ways: first, structures must be freestanding and, second, lots need to be platted in such a way so as to maximize the amount of sunlight that reaches each structure. These ideas were institutionalized during World War II, when model subdivision and health codes issued by the Federal Housing Administration (FHA) and professional societies included such recommendations.

Zoning for Health, Safety, and Welfare, 1907–1926

Zoning, a legal tool of local government to specify how land is to be used, forms an integral part of the story of the twentieth-century American city. From the time the basic idea arrived in the United States at the turn of the century, its proponents sold zoning as a way to improve the health of urban residents. To this day, health, safety, and welfare considerations underpin the legal basis for zoning, and zoning remains a powerful instrument for determining land use patterns by American municipalities.

Like the housing reformers, those who pressed for zoning in the first decades of the twentieth century built much of their case around public health issues. But unlike the housing reformers, the central goal of many zoning advocates was the protection of the physical health and the financial well-being of the upper and then, later, the middle classes, not the working and immigrant poor.[11] They wanted to create and protect the decentralized, decongested, leafy residential neighborhood, the healthy suburban environment that Olmsted had presaged several decades previously. To do so, they pushed for the adoption of codes that would keep out what they viewed as undesirable buildings and organizations—not just industrial operations but also structures that were far less offensive, including apartments and retail establishments of all kinds. Much of the motivation behind zoning stemmed from a desire, well-founded in the minds of its advocates, to ensure that America did not repeat its mistakes with respect to new housing on the suburban fringe. In their view, zoning would give planners the tool needed to control development, which would prevent the kinds of congestion and substandard housing that characterized the inner industrial city.[12]

Modern zoning is generally regarded to have begun in Germany toward the end of the nineteenth century. Concerned about rapid urban growth and development, German academics and municipal bureaucrats created the "districting" scheme, wherein entire cities would be differentiated by land uses and building types. The intent was to control and channel development brought about by industrialization, including the public health problems associated with pollution, overcrowding, and unsanitary environments. Advocates of the zoning idea in the United States adapted important aspects of German districting to the needs, as they saw them, of the American context. One critical change involved the degree of separation between residential, industrial, and commercial uses. In Germany, the districting system was never designed to completely separate uses. Frankfurt's ordinance contained mixed zones and even allowed for some nonresidential development in residential zones (Logan 1976). But American planners immediately began calling for a more rigid segregation of uses. For example, the Germans permitted apartments to be built over stores, a phenomenon that remains widespread in Europe today but has almost completely disappeared in the United States. American planners viewed such apartments with suspicion, strangely considering them to be a threat to public health and civic order (Williams 1913; Whitten 1921). In 1916, Veiller, who by this time had taken up a serious interest in zoning, claimed that retail stores themselves, including establishments as inoffensive as stationery shops, detracted from the enjoyment of residential neighborhoods and should be banished by zoning ordinances (Veiller 1916).

But the American proponents of zoning went even further, claiming that it was insufficient simply to create districts by type of use (residential, industrial, commercial). In their view, residential districts should be segregated by type of housing as well, insisting that some districts should consist entirely of single-family houses while others should contain only multifamily housing such as apartments. They asserted that apartments and tenements constituted qualitatively different types of housing than single-family homes, both in terms of the physical aspects of the structures themselves but also in terms of the type of residents they attracted. Leaders in real estate and related industries were often behind such views, calling for the public regulation of residential development in order to stabilize the housing market. In Los Angeles, for example, which led the nation in establishing the first zoning statute in a major city (1908), many members of these industries viewed zoning as a way to assuage the fears of upper-class homebuyers that their investments would not be eroded by the construction of multifamily housing in their neighborhoods (Weiss 1987). (The inequitable nature of zoning by class was hardly concealed by its proponents. Whitten once stated bluntly, "the protection of the homes of the people is probably the primary purpose of use districting" [Whitten 1918].) In New York, the city's Heights of Building Commission of 1913 contained many of the city's prominent minds in the fields of planning, law, housing, and commerce, including Whitten, Bassett, and Veiller, and would produce the report that led to New York's first zoning ordinance of 1916. While much of the commission's work focused on the problem of building heights in Manhattan, it also addressed the protection of the residential areas in the outer boroughs from the ravages—as they saw them—of the city, including the invasion of undesirable structures and people.

The arguments advanced by housing reformers to improve the tenement were now being used to confine the residents of such structures to the inner city. Zoning proponents consistently defended the neighborhood of single-family homes against encroachment by structures (and, by inference, of the people who inhabited these structures) deemed unacceptable by middle and upper-class residents (figure 2-1). In the same way that apartments and tenements needed to be designed and placed on the lot to increase the amount of sunlight and fresh air reaching the building, the reasoning went, houses also needed to be protected against apartments and tenements (Veiller 1916; Whitten 1918). In this view, apartments and tenements, and the renters who lived in them, represented a menace to the health and well-being of people who lived in single-family houses. Renters were believed to be less sanitary (Whitten 1921); their exclusion from single-family neighborhoods was claimed to increase family life and the safety and happiness of children (Bassett 1925; Hubbard and Hubbard 1929); and, it was argued, they detracted from the civic life of the community through the anticivic behaviors of the "renting class" (Whitten 1921) and by virtue of the physical crowding they created. "When families are crowded together in close proximity," stated the landscape architect and planner Henry Wright, "they seldom get acquainted one with another, and soon lose, or fail to develop, the neighborhood sense, and the neighborhood sense is the basis of responsible citizenship" (Wright 1913). Sentiments such as these led to calls for the outright prohibition of apartments in single-family housing developments and their subsequent concentration into high-density apartment districts (Whitten 1921).

Given the powerful sentiment for single-use, segregated zoning amongst planners, there was little standing in the way of the widespread implementation of zoning codes across the United States. As ordinances spread, zoning advocates quickly realized that zoning's constitutionality centered on whether restrictions could be placed on private property without compensation and whether zoning violated equal protection guarantees. Therefore, it can be argued that zoning amounted to a de facto segregation of cities into class- and race-based neighborhoods.

The zoning issue reached its legal zenith in 1926, when Justice George Sutherland delivered the majority opinion for the U.S. Supreme Court in the case of *Euclid versus Ambler Realty*. The village of Euclid, Ohio, a suburb of Cleveland, had passed a zoning ordinance that, like many others passed by municipalities around the country, mandated districts that would separate uses into residential and industrial categories and imposed height and bulk restrictions on the buildings erected in these districts. A firm, Ambler Realty, challenged the ordinance because, it argued, Euclid's residential zoning restrictions reduced the value of undeveloped property they had purchased within the city limits, and which they had intended to sell for industrial uses. The case revolved around the question of whether the ordinance was a constitutional use of the city's police power—its power to legislate for the health, safety, and welfare of its citizens. Briefs submitted on behalf of the city equated health with the residential district. The city's lawyer, for example, contrasted the "promised land" of the suburbs—where "fresh air and sunlight and a yard for children" could be found—with the "congested, accident producing, and smoke-filled condition of the city." Zoning, he asserted, was a tool the city needed to protect suburban dwellers' health, safety, and general welfare (Brooks 1989). The court in *Euclid* decided in support of the city's ordinance. In its decision, the majority framed two central questions, one a question of law and the other of fact. The central legal question concerned

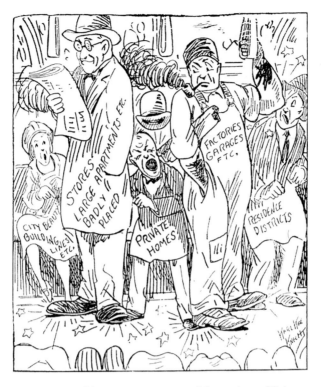

FIGURE 2-1. This cartoon was a part of the zoning publicity campaign in Evansville, Indiana, and appeared in the Evansville Courier and Journal in 1924. Source: Hubbard 1925.

whether it was constitutional for a municipality to create and maintain residential districts through zoning, "from which business and trade of every sort, including hotels and apartment houses, are excluded." The answer depended upon whether such restrictions could be interpreted as a reasonable exercise of the city's police power, "asserted for the public welfare." This argument set up the central factual question that was addressed in the decision, namely, whether Euclid's restrictions could be shown to have a "substantial relation to the public health, safety, morals, or general welfare." In the court's view, expert opinion had shown zoning's usefulness in preventing accidents by reducing traffic in residential districts; in decreasing the noise that intensified "nervous disorders"; and in preserving a "favorable environment in which to rear children." Moreover, the court observed, the building height and bulk restrictions contained in zoning ordinances prevented the construction of apartment buildings that interfered "by their height and bulk with the free circulation of air and [the monopoly of] the rays of the sun" (Beuscher, Wright, and Gitelman 1976).

The court had detailed the health and safety benefits of excluding apartments from single-family neighborhoods. While it accepted the argument that these restrictions contributed to the health and safety of people who lived in single-family homes in these neighborhoods, it did not address the question of whether people who lived in other types of neighborhoods would be subjected to a lower standard. In this respect its decision reflected the nature of the zoning argument advanced by its proponents, who undoubtedly believed that zoning would bring about more healthful conditions for those people who lived in the most favored residential zones. In their view, they were attempting to create a rational system by which residential neighborhoods could be protected from the urban conditions they defined as unhealthy and unsafe. The institutionalization of zoning in the 1920s thus laid the foundations on which today's cities have been built. The dominance of single-use development has its origins in the initial desire to separate commercial from residential uses. The preponderance of extremely low development densities in most American metropolitan regions is the result of the specification of maximum densities in zoning codes (through minimum lot size requirements), which in turn have their roots in the light-and-air thesis of early-twentieth-century zoning advocates. Finally, the economic segregation so characteristic of the American metropolis is a result, in part, of the wholesale exiling of apartment buildings from neighborhoods containing detached single-family homes.

Health and the Garden City, 1898–1930

As discussions over zoning intensified during the teens and twenties, a competing idea was making its mark on the thinking of American planners. In many respects, this idea, the garden city, was a genuine alternative to the standard suburban model of the time, which consisted of satellite suburbs arrayed around a central city. In contrast, this vision called for a number of small, freestanding cities dotting the regional landscape, each separated by wide greenbelts of farms or forests. Each city would be large enough to provide residents with the advantages of urban life (civic life, employment opportunities, culture) but small enough to provide the fruits of rural living, which for the most part consisted of the health benefits that access to nature provides. Yet, for all of this movement's radicalism, it did not deviate from some of the standard assumptions about how to solve urban health problems.

In 1902, an Englishman, Ebenezer Howard, formulated the original garden city concept in his famous treatise on the subject, *Garden Cities of Tomorrow*.[13] As with many others imbued with reformist zeal during this period, Howard viewed the modern city, in particular London, as overcrowded, dirty, and unhealthy—"ulcers on the very face of our beautiful island" (Howard 1946, 145). Rejecting the modern industrial city as unworkable, Howard believed that human needs and aspirations could best be met through a new type of settlement that combined the best elements of both city and countryside, and that such cities could be created only through a new set of social and economic relationships. Howard possessed a radical vision for the restructuring of the bases of his society. To finance and build his cities, he proposed to create a limited-dividend company that would buy the land and finance the houses. Residents would pay off their cottages to a fund that would be used to establish a local welfare state, which among other things would provide for old-age pensions. Citizens would be self-governing, running their municipality themselves and sharing in its fiscal and social dividends. These elements of Howard's original vision, while not copied exactly, nonetheless would inspire later advocates of the garden city in both Europe and the United States (Hall 1996).

Howard's most enduring legacy, and the one for which he is best remembered, consists of his plans for the physical layout of his garden cities. He envisioned a polycentric network of cities, each built with public funds on about 6,000 acres of rural land located well outside of existing urban centers, large enough for perhaps 30,000 residents. The street network of each city would consist of a simple spoke-and-wheel pattern, with the main institutional buildings at the center of the wheel, housing in the middle, and factories on the outskirts. Each city would contain its own civic, educational, cultural, and recreational facilities. Housing would be in the form of detached cottages. The cities would provide for employment of their residents via factories located in the town, close enough for an easy walk from home to work. Most importantly, each city would be surrounded by large greenbelts of agricultural land that would be preserved in perpetuity. The greenbelts would serve to prevent existing cities from encroaching upon the new town (thereby destroying the latter's character) as well as the garden cities from overrunning each other. They would, further, provide residents with easy access to nature. Finally, inter-city rail would transport goods and passengers between all of the cities (figure 2-2).

Howard clearly viewed nature as a source of physical, psychological, and mental health. Nature's health benefits, in fact, underpinned much of Howard's argument for the garden city. Howard's goal was to construct "a healthy, natural, and economic combination of town and country life" (Howard 1946, 51). In his famous "Three Magnets" drawing (figure 2-3), the "Town-Country" magnet—the garden city—married the best of the town (social opportunity, high wages, flow of capital) with those of the country (beauty of nature, pure air and water, no smoke, no slums). By surrounding his towns with the countryside, "with its canopy of sky, the air that blows upon it, the sun that warms it, the rain and dew that moisten it," Howard believed his cities would "pour a flood of light" onto the problems of his age, which he defined as including intemperance, overwork, anxiety, and poverty (Howard 1946, 44). By providing a municipally owned greenbelt around the city, "the free gifts of Nature—fresh air, sunlight, breathing room and playing room—[would be] retained in all needed abundance" (Howard 1946, 127).

The garden city idea spread rapidly, reaching the United States early in the new century, where its devotees could be found in a diverse array of fields, most notably in city planning. But the conservatism of many planners during the period meant that serious calls for the creation of garden cities would have to wait until the formation of the Regional Planning Association of America (RPAA) in 1923 (Buder 1990). The RPAA consisted of a small number of intellectuals who were interested in radical approaches to solving urban as well as rural problems. RPAA members included some of the most important people in the history of American planning, architecture, housing, and economics: Lewis Mumford, Benton MacKaye, Henry Wright, Clarence Stein, Stuart Chase, Clarence Perry, Charles Harris Whitaker, and Catherine Wurster (Christensen 1986). The RPAA, as Mumford would later describe it, was dedicated to "the building of balanced communities, cut to human scale, in balanced regions, which would be part of an ever widening national, continental, and global whole, also in balance" (quotation in Schaffer 1982, 55).

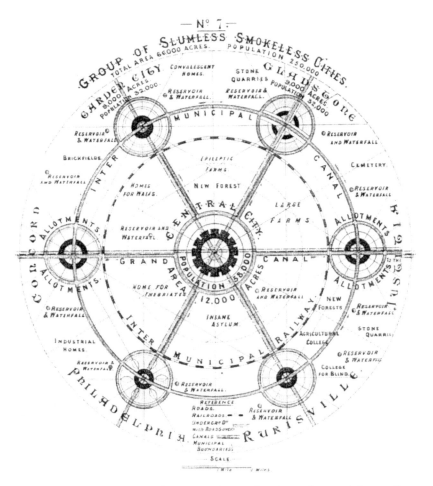

FIGURE 2-2. Ebenezer Howard's diagram showing his vision of regional decentralization. His call for garden cities surrounded by greenbelts and connected to each other and the central city had a powerful influence on both sides of the Atlantic. Source: Howard 1946.

While it was thus formed in order to advance multiple causes, including affordable housing, at the RPAA's center stood a commitment to polynucleated development based on the garden city model (Schaffer 1982). Individual members of the RPAA readily admitted to their fascination with Howard's ideas. Stein and Wright traveled to England specifically to tour the garden city of Letchworth, built by Howard's disciple Raymond Unwin, and to discuss design issues with both of them (Lubove 1963). Mumford showed his

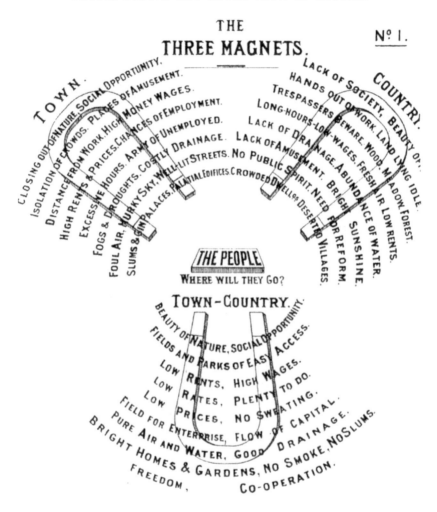

FIGURE 2-3. Ebenezer Howard's "Three Magnets" drawing. The message is clear: health and prosperity will result from a marriage of city and country. Source: Howard 1946.

commitment to the garden city ideal when he strongly criticized New York's regional plan of 1931, the result of years of effort by that region's top municipal planners; he viewed it as being hugely inadequate because it did not fulfill the basic principles for regional development as outlined by Howard. Mumford said that the plan "talks garden cities but drifts toward further metropolitan centralization" and criticized it for placing new suburban development within the city's existing suburban boundary, "instead of in the cheaper agricultural areas beyond" (Mumford 1932, 122–3), echoing Howard's call for placing garden cities in rural areas.

Spatially, RPAA members wanted to build garden cities well outside of existing metropolitan areas in order to take advantage of cheap land; in so doing, the capital that was saved could be redirected to housing design and construction. Like Howard, they believed that the provision of high quality but inexpensive housing for the masses would require fundamental changes in economic and spatial relationships. Economically, they wanted to dampen or eliminate the speculative building process that they viewed as inflating housing costs. As Howard had been, they were driven toward this position by a basic distrust of the market and its ability to deliver quality, low-cost housing without government intervention (Buder 1990; Schaffer 1982; Lubove 1963).

The RPAA never succeeded in building a true garden city, in large part because the organization was not dedicated to the actual construction of such a development. But individual members did attempt to apply these ideas to real projects, with the full knowledge and cooperation of the larger organization (Christensen 1986). The most famous of these were Sunnyside Gardens, in Queens, and Radburn in New Jersey and both planned by Stein and Wright. Sunnyside and Radburn were attempts to rectify what Stein viewed as a long list of physical and mental ills that resulted from living in the modern city: strained nerves, tension, physical disabilities, declining birthrate, breakdown, madness, life and movement imprisoned by the grid, "death at every street crossing" for pedestrians, "sunless, insanitary [sic], filthy, congested slums," packed buses and subways, automobile congestion, blocked sunlight and breezes, loneliness, lack of community, separation from nature, wasted time, and development made ugly by "monotonous regimentation, smoke, and dirt" (Stein 1957). Sunnyside Gardens was begun in 1924 and consisted of 1,200 housing units—mostly apartments—on a 55-acre site. Wright later described Sunnyside as a "laboratory" for testing the RPAA's main ideas in planning and building affordable housing. The objective was to prove that low cost housing could be built along with amenities for residents, such as open spaces for recreation and leisure. While Stein was reasonably happy with his experiment—Mumford would later move into one of the apartments—he felt the design was hampered by constraints imposed on the project from outside. For one thing, the site was located near existing development, meaning that it did not follow the garden city ideal of countryside living. For another, development had to occur within the constraints imposed by an existing grid street system, a fact that greatly annoyed the architects (Stein 1957).

Radburn, begun in 1929, attempted to rectify many of these problems. Locating their new community on a large tract of farmland, Stein and Wright aimed to build three neighborhoods housing about 25,000 people. Radburn did not approximate a "pure" garden city because space limitations prevented its designers from surrounding it with a greenbelt. However, Stein still considered Radburn to be a dramatic improvement upon Sunnyside, believing that it constituted a "new form of city and community." Radburn's design was in some ways brand new, anticipating postwar subdivision design. Its layout reflected Stein's unhappiness with traditional street layouts, namely the grid pattern that had hindered Stein's freedom of action in Sunnyside. In the grid's place, Stein and Wright created a dendritic network of streets, with major, secondary, and tertiary roads (for a lengthy discussion of street networks, see chapter 7). They also separated automobile from pedestrian traffic in order to enhance pedestrian safety. Finally, they turned the entire development's focus inward onto itself, rather than outward to the street, through two principal design treatments: they created a series of small parks in between rows of houses, and turned the houses around to face the parks rather than the streets on which the houses were located. This turned the parks, Stein later wrote, into Radburn's backbone (Stein 1957).

Stein and Wright placed great emphasis upon the significance of the car for urban form. The Radburn plan thus became one of the first to be designed specifically with the automobile in mind. Urban planners had been busy facilitating the explosive growth of automobile travel during the 1920s, constructing freeways, widening streets, rounding corners at intersections, and ignoring the infrastructure for other modes of travel, including transit and pathways for pedestrians and bicyclists (Fairfield 1994).[14] To Stein, this growth in auto use meant that the traditional street layout, the grid pattern, was "as obsolete as a fortified town wall." As he saw the problem, the grid required frequent street crossings for pedestrians, jeopardizing their safety. As the grid's high connectivity meant that every street was a through street, child safety was also jeopardized because, as Stein saw it, the roadbed was the primary playground for most children living in cities (Stein 1957). Hence Stein and Wright's desire to control the ravages of the automobile on residential neighborhoods: to prevent injury, a thorough rethinking of the street was needed in terms of its layout and function. They sought to prevent motorists from driving through the neighborhood at high speeds. This was accomplished through disconnecting the neighborhood's street network from the larger city beyond the neighborhood's boundaries; the Radburn network consisted of multiple cul-de-sacs, making it impossible to travel directly across the neighborhood by car.

One inspiration for Radburn's street design was a concept articulated by the planner Clarence Perry in 1923. Perry had a longstanding interest in community recreation issues, work that had involved him in Progressive causes before World War I. During the 1920s, Perry became loosely affiliated with the RPAA, and presented his basic idea for urban design, the Neighborhood Unit Plan, to that group. RPAA members, including Mumford and Stein, received his idea with much enthusiasm, and the RPAA later endorsed the concept of neighborhood planning as the basis for a national housing policy (Gillette 1983). Perry's concept was based on the premise that the neighborhood is the basic unit around which the city should be designed. Perry agreed with Stein and Wright that the car had changed the urban equation on a fundamental level. Traffic thoroughfares were revolutionizing the city's form by cleaving existing neighborhoods in half, creating islands that were isolated from one another and from the fabric of the larger city. It was into these gaps created by the thoroughfares that Perry believed planners had to turn their attention. "Arterial highways," he argued, "must necessarily run in every direction and turn the street system into a network, and that residential life must occupy the interstitial spaces" (Perry 1929). It was no longer feasible to design cities according to a citywide model. The car had made the "interstitial spaces"— neighborhoods—the only units that could be controlled for planning purposes. It was here, he was saying, that the health and well-being of the city's residents lay.

Perry believed the neighborhood had four functions: education (schools), recreational space for children (playgrounds), service provision (shops), and a safe, attractive environment (neighborhood character). The spatial boundaries of Perry's neighborhood "units" were defined by the first two functions: a unit should be sized so that children did not have to cross any arterial to reach a playground or a schoolyard, and within walking distance of both. Each unit was to be roughly a half-mile on a side, have a school and playground at the center, have narrow, curvilinear interior roadways and be bounded by major roads on all sides (figure 2-4). The interior roadways were narrow and disconnected to facilitate intra-neighborhood pedestrian travel while discouraging through-traffic. Meanwhile, the roads that bounded the neighborhood on all sides not only encouraged traffic to bypass the neighborhood entirely, but also were deliberately intended to assist in isolating the neighborhood from outsiders, ensuring its social cohesiveness. Perry called the arterials the "walls of our protected cell," signifying his desire to isolate the neighborhood as much as possible from the outside (Perry 1929, 52).

The garden city movement placed social, economic, and personal well-being at the center of its agenda. While there were only a few attempts at constructing garden cities or "garden suburbs" in the United States, including the aforementioned Sunnyside and Radburn as well as later versions of the same thing (the New Deal greenbelt program and the New Towns movement of the 1960s), the garden city movement represented an attempt to create a genuine alternative to the standard suburb. Its advocates believed that garden cities would be true communities that would fight residents' alienation from each other and from their surroundings (Allen 1977). However, in terms of public health, the garden city position was very much within the orthodox mainstream: sunshine, fresh air, outdoor recreation, proximity to nature, and sanitation were the end states of the garden city. Moreover, as illustrated by the designs of Stein, Wright, and Perry, the garden city movement helped to further the idea of the self-contained neighborhood. By seeking design solutions that focused on the neighborhood interior instead of the larger urban context, they helped to create and institutionalize the ideal of the detached subdivision in American city planning, separated one from another by major roadways (Wolfe 1987). It is true that had Howard's original design proposals been faithfully adopted, we likely would have communities much more oriented toward nonmotorized transportation than we have today. A similar conclusion might be warranted in Perry's case, although his design was intended to maximize walking within the boundaries of the neighborhood while minimizing inter-neighborhood contact. Nonetheless, Perry sought to disconnect the neighborhood from the city, adapting streets to the use they "are destined to have" (Perry 1929, 85). Stein wanted to separate entirely the nonmotorist from the motorist and turn buildings around from the roadway to face

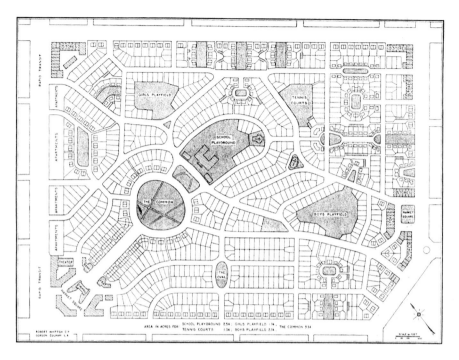

FIGURE 2-4. Clarence Perry's Neighborhood Unit Plan was based upon the idea that the city needed to be broken down into self-contained neighborhoods. Perry made use of this drawing, created by Robert Whitten, to illustrate the idea. Motorists were discouraged from passing through the neighborhood by the lack of direct routes from one side to the other, while the use of major roads on all four sides was intended to discourage nonresident pedestrians from accessing the neighborhood. Source: Robert Whitten, "A 160-Acre Neighborhood Unit Subdivision." In *Housing for the Machine Age,* by Clarence Arthur Perry. Copyright 1939 Russell Sage Foundation, 112 East 64th Street, New York, NY, 10021. Reprinted with permission.

interior courtyards, in the process diminishing the critical role played by streets in urban design and turning them into mere pathways for cars (this is discussed more thoroughly in chapter 9). Therefore, despite the fact that this group ultimately lost out in determining the direction of suburban growth in the United States, it can be fairly claimed that they contributed to the cementation of the idea that the good city, the healthful city, is decentralized, decongested, and disconnected.

Conclusion

This chapter has shown that public health was a motive force in determining the thinking of those professionals who shaped the industrial city during the nineteenth and early twentieth centuries. Public health concerns were uppermost in the minds of leading figures in fields as diverse as urban planning, architecture, housing, real estate, engineering, and landscape architecture as members of these professions envisioned, and then sought to implement, solutions to the problems that beset the industrial city. By the middle of the last century, these reformers had won a total victory and had created or rewritten the basic ground rules by which all cities in the United States would be built over the subsequent decades. After the Second World War, a few voices in planning and architectural circles expressed their dismay with the suburban consensus that had risen to dominance and that was beginning the process, by the 1950s, of utterly transforming the face of the country. Some, such as the urbanist William Whyte and the architectural critic Jane Jacobs, both of whom are now considered luminaries in their fields, engaged in a ferocious rearguard action against both suburban growth and the decline of the urban core.[15] Yet despite the intellectual and emotional doubts of a few intellectuals and academics, the onward march of suburbia as a real, on-the-ground solution to a variety of urban problems has continued unabated down to the present. Therefore, nearly all new development in the United States is being driven, in a sense, by the public health problems of a century and more ago. Meanwhile, the public health picture has changed considerably, both in terms of our understanding of the causes as well as the solutions to our ever changing tableau of health challenges. In 1900, the leading causes of death were infectious and communicable diseases such as pneumonia and tuberculosis. Now, the leading causes of death are noncommunicable diseases caused not by bacterial or viral infection but by routine behavior and related daily habits. Ironically, the urban solutions that were implemented decades ago to help solve public health problems of the day now contribute to these health risks and the onset of chronic disease. Tools such as zoning that were developed during the early twentieth century provided planners with a "police power" to control growth for the promotion of the health, safety, and welfare of the public. However, the evolution of such development regulations into legal prescriptions for auto-dependent and sprawling environments highlights a widening divergence between their intent and an important consequence, namely, physical inactivity.

CHAPTER THREE

Physical Activity and Public Health

All parts of the body which were made for active use, if moderately used and exercised at the labor to which they are habituated, become healthy, increase in bulk, and bear their age well, but when not used, and when left without exercise, they become diseased, their growth is arrested, and they soon become old."

HIPPOCRATES,
On the Articulations (ca. 460–377 B.C.)

The prevention and cure of many infectious diseases, due in large part to advances in medical science as well as widespread improvements in sanitation, diet, and housing, was a contributing factor in the dramatic increase in longevity between the beginning and end of the twentieth century. In 1900, the average American could expect to live to age forty-nine; by 1997, this figure was around seventy-six years (Federal Interagency Forum on Aging-Related Statistics 2000). Obviously, the public health issues facing Americans and residents of other wealthy countries have changed in dramatic ways. Certainly, the suffering and premature deaths that used to accompany infectious disease epidemics are now rare. However, hundreds of thousands of Americans still die from *preventable* deaths each year. Deaths from chronic diseases, most notably heart disease and various cancers, have replaced deaths from infectious disease. Many deaths from the sources listed in figure 3-1 can be traced to bad habits. They are preventable in that they are mostly caused by behaviors that can be modified; smoking, for example, is a well-known cause of lung cancer. But premature mortality is not the only consequence of preventable medical problems. Chronic diseases and other preventable afflictions also subtract from one's quality of life. For instance, osteoporosis, a condition that tends to affect many older women, is characterized by a deterioration in one's bone mass and structure; the onset of osteoporosis may be delayed or prevented by modifiable behaviors, for example dietary and exercise patterns.

Unfortunately, Americans engage in many different behaviors that lead to such ill health. Physical inactivity is one of the most common and most preventable patterns of behavior. In this chapter we describe how this widespread inactivity is a major determinant of poor health in the general population, in terms of premature mortality, the onset of chronic diseases, and a poor quality of life. Physical activity can be a significant part of the solution to many of these health problems. Recent public health research has shown that moderate forms of physical activity can be helpful types of exercise. While more vigorous forms of activity such as running can generate health benefits for participants, from a public health perspective it may be better to focus on moderate types of physical activity because they are easier for inactive people to begin and maintain over time. Moderately intense activities can be built into the lives of many Americans by changing the way communities are designed and built. Two of the most common types, walking and bicycling, are easily incorporated into people's lives when the built environment is properly structured to encourage them. However, when our communities are structured so that they inhibit or prevent such activities, as is the case in most parts of the country, many people are unable to get the amount of physical activity needed for long-term health.

Physical Activity and Health: Basic Premises

While it has long been known that physical activity is an important component of a healthy lifestyle, a report issued by the Surgeon General in 1996 titled *Physical Activity and Health* represented a watershed moment in the history of the public health community's approach to physical activity and fitness (U.S. Department of Health and Human Services 1996, hereafter USD-HHS 1996). Prior to this report, the general advice given by public health officials to the public was echoed in the phrase "no pain—no gain," whereby individuals were advised to try and get at least twenty minutes of high intensity

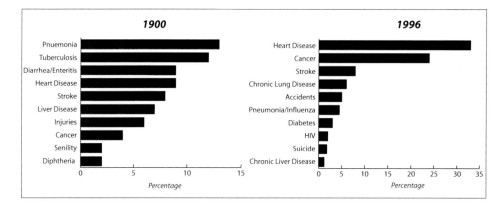

FIGURE 3-1. The ten leading proximate causes of deaths (as a percentage of all deaths) per year in the United States, 1900 and 1996. Source: Centers for Disease Control, National Center for Health Statistics.

aerobic exercise three or more days a week (Pate et al. 1995). Implicit in this advice was the idea that anything less than a sustained high-energy effort would be a waste of time, resulting in little or no health improvement over time. While the Surgeon General's report recognized the benefits of the increased fitness that vigorous exercise can provide, it took a much more inclusive view of physical activity and health. In a nutshell, it voiced the expert opinion, based upon an exhaustive reading of recent health research, that significant health benefits can be obtained through moderate activities such as walking and bicycling. These new recommendations are for adults to accumulate at least thirty minutes of moderate physical activity on most, preferably each day of the week.

Since the publication of the Surgeon General's report, the body of scientific literature that supports this position has continued to grow. Regular, moderately intense physical activity helps to maintain the functional independence of older adults and enhances the quality of life for people of all ages. The literature also shows that such physical activity helps maintain normal muscle strength and joint structure and function, lower high blood pressure, relieve depression and anxiety, lower obesity levels, and is necessary for normal skeletal development during childhood. Physically inactive people are almost twice as likely to develop coronary heart disease as people who engage in regular physical activity. This risk is almost as high as several well-known risk factors such as cigarette smoking, high blood pressure and high cholesterol. Sadly, however, physical inactivity in the United States is more common than any of these other major risk factors, with different studies showing that the majority of Americans do not get enough physical activity to meet minimum standards set by the Surgeon General and other health organizations (USDHHS 1996). While a lifetime of regular physical activity is the goal, it is never too late to start. In fact when sedentary people become more active they gain immediate health benefits, often with a larger relative improvement than their more fit counterparts. As shown in figure 3-2, the marginal benefits that result from a unit increase in physical activity for the sedentary person is thought to be larger than the same increase would be for the person who is already a committed runner or soccer player.

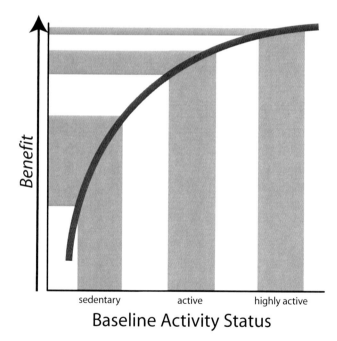

Baseline Activity Status

FIGURE 3-2. Marginal health benefit of exercise. Source: Pate et al., "Physical activity and health: A recommendation from the Centers for Disease Control and Prevention and the American College of Sports Medicine," *Journal of the American Medical Association*, 1995, Vol. 273, No. 5, 402–407.

The Price of Inactivity

While genetics provide an important contribution to longevity, daily habits may play an even more critical role in determining life expectancy. Epidemiological studies have consistently linked physical inactivity to mortality over the long run. Based upon statistical evidence, these studies generally show that individuals with higher physical activity levels experience lower mortality rates. One found, for example, that men who engaged in moderate physical activity had a risk of dying that was only 73 percent of that for the least active group of men in the study (Leon et al. 1987). Another study concluded that slight improvements in fitness can have a dramatic effect on long-term mortality risk (Blair et al. 1989).

Other studies have yielded similar findings, even after controlling for the influence of one's genetics (Paffenbarger and Lee 1996). In an effort to isolate the influence of physical activity patterns on mortality while taking genetics into account, Kujala et al. (1998) examined the relationship between exercise patterns and mortality in about 19,000 subjects who shared the same childhood environments and nearly identical genetic structure. The researchers tracked the health status of the subjects over a twenty-year period. The results showed that the risk of death declined with increasing physical activity in both men and women, even after genetic and other familial variables are taken into account.

Studies such as this one have contributed to an expanded interest, within public health circles, regarding how "behavioral risk factors" (e.g., smoking, poor diet, inadequate physical activity) influence health and mortality. Hundreds of thousands of premature deaths per year can be attributed to poor diet and inadequate levels of physical activity. One study estimated the number of deaths attributable to poor dietary and physical activity patterns in the United States in 1990 (McGinnis and Foege 1993). The authors' goal was to assess the role played by underlying behaviors (tobacco use, poor diet and activity patterns, alcohol abuse, etc.) instead of the immediate health conditions that caused death (lung disease, emphysema, diabetes, heart disease, etc.), which were seen as the result of risky behavior. The authors reviewed studies published between 1977 and 1993 of the causes of death in different study populations, allowing them to derive approximations of the number of deaths in the United States that could be assigned to underlying behavior. The data in table 3-1 represent the authors' best estimates of the number of deaths attributable to each root cause. Poor diet and sedentary living patterns, estimated to have caused some 300,000 deaths (14 percent of all deaths), ranked as the second leading cause, behind tobacco but ahead of such well-known causes as firearms and motor vehicle accidents.

PHYSICAL INACTIVITY AND CHRONIC DISEASE

Chronic diseases and mortality are, of course, intimately linked. National and international health organizations, for example the Centers for Disease Control and Prevention (CDC) in the United States, believe that long-term patterns of behaviors—in particular, tobacco use, poor nutrition, and lack of physical activity—play significant roles in the onset of four main chronic diseases (cardiovascular disease, cancer, diabetes, and chronic obstructive pulmonary disease) and, thus, in premature mortality (CDC 1999a). In a study of data from national health surveys, the CDC determined that a sedentary lifestyle was the most common modifiable risk factor for coronary heart disease (CHD, a form of cardiovascular disease), present in 58 percent of reported cases. In contrast, cigarette smoking was present 25 percent of the time, obesity 22 percent, and hypertension 17 percent (CDC 1990). Physical inactivity also has been linked to the other chronic diseases. The Surgeon General's 1996 report concluded that physical inactivity is associated with an increased risk of colon cancer and diabetes (USDHHS 1996). Other studies have addressed walking as a predictor of diabetes. One compared the activity patterns with the risk of becoming diabetic for women over a period of eight years; those who walked frequently had only 58 percent of the risk of becoming diabetic when compared with sedentary women, even after controlling for age, hypertension, and other variables (Hu et al. 1999).

There is enormous potential for physical activity to reduce the amount of chronic disease in the United States. One study (Powell and Blair 1994), found that between 32 percent and 35 percent of deaths attributable to CHD, colon cancer, and diabetes could have been prevented if every person in the United States were to become highly active. The authors of this study, realizing that it would be unlikely for all people in the country to be active at this level, also generated estimates based on smaller improvements in physical activity rates within the population. Modest improvements in physical activity levels, they

TABLE 3-1
Actual causes of death in the United States, 1990

Causes	Deaths	
	Estimated number*	Percentage of total deaths
Tobacco	400,000	19
Diet/activity patterns	300,000	14
Alcohol	100,000	5
Microbial agents	90,000	4
Toxic agents	60,000	3
Firearms	35,000	2
Sexual behavior	30,000	1
Motor vehicles	25,000	1
Illicit drug use	20,000	<1
Total	1,060,000	50

*See text for discussion of the distinction between underlying causes of death and proximate or immediate causes.

SOURCE: J. Michael McGinnis and William Foege, "Actual causes of death in the United States," *Journal of the American Medical Association*, 1993, Vol. 270, No. 18, pp. 2207–2212.

estimated, would still result in substantial reductions in deaths attributable to the three diseases because of the huge numbers of people who fall into the inactive categories. For example, if half of the population classified as sedentary were to become irregularly active (meaning getting some activity but not enough to meet guidelines), the total number of deaths attributable to CHD, colon cancer, and diabetes would drop 3.9 percent, 2.5 percent, and 1.5 percent, respectively. If half of the people who are irregularly active were to become regularly active (thus meeting the guidelines), those figures would be 7.1 percent, 7.4 percent, and 5.2 percent. This study illustrates the public health principle of obtaining large population benefits from small average individual change. A few percentage points' improvement in the national average for blood pressure, or a few minutes added to the national average of daily exercise would result in a large number of saved lives.

PHYSICAL INACTIVITY: OVERWEIGHT AND OBESITY

In the United States, rising overweight and obesity is a serious public health problem. "Overweight" and "obesity" are clinical terms used by public health agencies that classify people according to their height and weight status; the overweight category is one category above normal (heavier than normal for one's height), while the obese category is yet another category above overweight.[1] Unfortunately, more than half of American adults are categorized as being overweight or obese. A national study of CDC data reported that in 1999–2000 nearly one-third (30.5 percent) of adults were obese and nearly two-thirds (64.5 percent) were overweight or obese (Flegal et al. 2002). To make matters worse, levels of overweight and obesity have been climbing for many years. Roughly speaking, the prevalence of obesity in the United States increased by 61 percent during the 1990s alone. This trend appears to be affecting all major demographic groups in society. Rising overweight and obesity is pervasive and widespread in the United States, affecting the young and old, black and white, rich and poor. To illustrate, the maps in figure 3-3 show both the rapid increase in obesity over time as well as the extent of the problem in the United States (Mokdad et al. 2001). Levels of childhood obesity are similarly worrisome. In the 1960s and 1970s about 4 to 6 percent of children and adolescents (ages 6–19) were overweight; by 1999, this number had more than doubled to 13–14 percent (CDC 1999d). Overall, the rate of increase of obesity in the American population—about 50 percent during the 1990s—is considered so severe that many have compared its spread and dispersion characteristics to that of a communicable disease epidemic (Mokdad et al. 1999).[2]

Overweight and obesity have been linked in the public health literature to a variety of diseases and health problems. Overweight and obesity are associated with high blood pressure, gallbladder disease, osteoarthritis, and type 2 diabetes mellitus, relationships that get stronger as a person gets heavier. These findings are consistent for both men and women. Further, as a person's weight increases their chance of having two or more of these chronic conditions multiplies (Must et al. 1999).

While physical inactivity by itself does not generally cause overweight and obesity, the combination of sedentary lifestyles with other risk behaviors such as improper diet leads to these conditions. Only some of the increase in overweight and obesity rates can be explained by the increases in average caloric intake over time for the American population; low and declining levels of physical activity are also assumed to be a significant contributor (Koplan and Dietz 2000). The Surgeon General's report, for example, subscribes to the formulation that dietary patterns plus exercise are important determinants of overweight and obesity in the United States (USDHHS 1996; see also Must et al. 1999). Numerous cross-sectional studies reviewed by the Surgeon General reported lower weight among people with higher levels of physical activity.

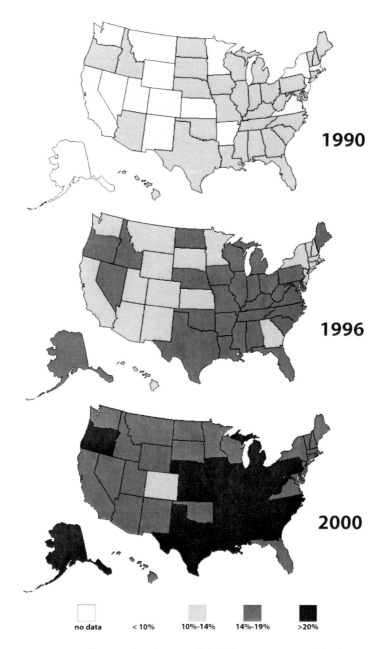

FIGURE 3-3. Percent obese by state, United States, 1990–2000. Absolute figures vary from sources quoted in the text due to different survey methodologies. Source: Mokdad et al. 2001. Original data from the Behavioral Risk Factor Surveillance System (BRFSS).

The Surgeon General's report concluded that: physical activity promotes fat loss while preserving or increasing lean mass; the rate of weight loss is associated with the frequency and duration of physical activity; the combination of increased physical activity and dieting is more effective than dieting alone for long-term weight regulation; and the full extent that physical inactivity contributes to obesity levels in children is not yet determined.

PHYSICAL INACTIVITY AND QUALITY OF LIFE

Regular physical activity has a large number of benefits beyond those of reducing the risk of chronic disease and premature mortality. Physical activity maintains muscle strength, bone mass, and proper joint function and may also play an important role in fostering and maintaining mental health. People may have a more positive self-evaluation of their physical and mental status if they are more active, a phenomenon that becomes more prevalent as they get older (Unger 1995).

A lifetime of physical activity may, in fact, generate its greatest benefits for the elderly. A recent analysis of elderly women, for example, reported that inactive, nonsmoking women at age sixty-five have 12.7 years of active life expectancy, compared to 18.4 years of active life expectancy for more highly active women (Ferucci et al. 2000). Because physical activity is believed to delay the onset of disability and chronic diseases, the functional limitations and subsequent loss of independence that are associated with aging are also delayed. Physical activity is believed to be able to help delay or prevent the onset of osteoporosis in the elderly, a condition characterized by decreased bone mass and increased bone fragility. This is a particularly severe problem in older women, contributing to the widespread and growing number of hip fractures from falls. Regular physical activity throughout one's life may prevent or delay the development of osteoporosis, particularly by helping to develop and maintain bone mass during adolescence and middle age (USD-HHS 1996; Shephard 1997). Many studies also demonstrate that physical activity improves symptoms of depression in adults. One study found that exercise programs for adults produced improvements in depressive symptoms that were comparable to improvements from medication (Singh, Clemets, and Fiatarone 1997), while another reported that physical activity for adults reduces the amount of cognitive decline as an adult ages (Yaffe et al. 2001). The benefits of exercise are not limited to improvements in cognitive function. A Boston study of forty- to seventy-year-old men found that physical activity status was significantly associated with erectile dysfunction (impotence). The highest risk was for men who remained inactive, and the lowest was among those who remained active or became physically active, even if begun at middle age (Derby et al. 2000).

ECONOMIC COST OF PHYSICAL INACTIVITY

Premature death and disability caused by coronary heart disease, diabetes mellitus, cancers, and other illnesses related to physical inactivity result in tremendous health care costs. According to the American Heart Association, cardiovascular disease costs the country more than $150 billion each year in direct and indirect costs, including hospital and nursing home services, prescription drugs, and lost productivity (Stone 1996). Studies that have examined the results of one of the most thorough national surveys of medical expenditures, the National Medical Expenditure Survey, report lower direct medical costs for people who are active versus those who are sedentary. Annual medical costs remained lower for the regularly active group (ranging from $330 to more than $1,000 per person), even after controlling for the independent influence of physical limitations, gender, and smoking status. These findings also applied to particular types of health care costs. For example, direct health care costs for treatment of people who had arthritis were found to be about $1,200 less for those who were physically active than those who were sedentary (Pratt, Macera, and Wang 2000; Wang et al. 2001).

Levels of Physical Inactivity

A minority of the American population engages in enough regular, sustained exercise to meet public health recommendations. Data released by the CDC in 2001 from the Behavorial Risk Factor Surveillance System (BRFSS) showed that in 2000 only about one out of three adults reported enough moderate or vigorous activity to meet public health guidelines while a similar number (29%) were sedentary—reporting no leisure time physical activity. The remainder (about 46%) reported some activity but at a level insufficient to maintain personal health and wellness. As shown in figure 3-4 these patterns of leisure time activity have remained essentially stable since the 1980s (CDC 2001b).

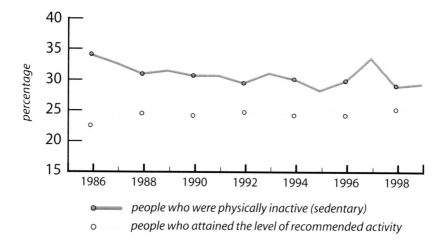

FIGURE 3-4. Leisure time physical activity trends, United States, 1986–1999. Source: Data provided by Sandra Ham, Centers for Disease Control and Prevention, and adapted from CDC 2001b.

Poor physical activity habits typically start at a young age. Among high school students more than one in three (35 percent) do not participate regularly in vigorous physical activity. Regular participation drops from 75 percent of ninth graders to 61 percent of twelfth graders. From 1991 to 2001 participation in daily physical education classes in high school dropped from 42 percent to 31 percent of students. Overall about one in three (31 percent) students do not meet minimum guidelines for physical activity (Grunbaum et al. 2002). Unfortunately, there is evidence that such bad habits persist into adulthood. Studies in the United States and Europe have found that there is a moderate to low correlation between activity levels in childhood and later as adults. Children who are inactive are more likely to be inactive when they are adults than their active peers (Malina 2001; Telama et al. 1997). Physical activity patterns also vary by other demographic and socioeconomic patterns. Rates of physical activity are lower for females than males, generally lower for minorities, the elderly, the less educated, and the poor, and declines with age.

Encouraging Physical Activity: Adoption and Adherence

One of the flaws in the "no pain—no gain" model of physical activity outlined at the beginning of this chapter is that people may have a difficult time beginning the types of exercise that this model prescribes and, further, an even more difficult time in sticking to such exercise routines over longer terms. Public health research often centers on these phenomena—called adoption (beginning a physical activity regimen) and adherence (sticking to one over time)—because they are important concepts in explaining why people have problems altering their physical activity patterns. Given the findings of the Surgeon General and others that significant health benefits for an individual can be achieved via thirty minutes or more of moderate physical activity, which can be accumulated throughout the course of the day in short bouts (i.e., in as little as ten minutes at a time), attention has been focused on the question of whether people can more readily adopt and adhere to these forms of physical activity. Sustained participation in structured activities (the gym-based model of exercise) has proven to be very difficult to achieve for many people. In contrast, there is some evidence to suggest that unstructured activities (where people do not have to join a gym or other structured, formal setting) of moderate intensity may be more effective. While structured exercise programs may have a slightly greater effect on health than unstructured activities *per unit of time,* the latter type may be better for many people because it is easier to get people to adopt and adhere to them (Dunn, Andersen, and Jakicic 1998).

Some health educators use the term "lifestyle" to denote that patterns of some behaviors are good predictors of other behaviors—that is, people who tend to be careful about what they eat also may be careful about getting enough physical activity (or, conversely, if people have some bad habits such as smoking or taking illegal drugs they may be less concerned about an unhealthy diet or abuse of alcohol).

While this approach has value for those in the field of public health who design health promotion programs, it is less salient for our purposes than a second meaning of the term. Within the context of physical activity research, lifestyle activities are those that can fit easily into one's daily routine. For instance, riding a bicycle to the store may be an easier habit to establish and maintain than finding the extra time to go to the gym and work out. This stands in contrast to traditional exercises that are, as the kinesiologist William Morgan has written, nonpurposeful and therefore have little meaning in and of themselves. (Morgan quotes the Roman poet Marcus Valerius Martialis [A.D. 38–103] in this context, who asked, "Why do strong arms fatigue themselves with frivolous dumbbells? To dig in a vineyard is worthier exercise for men." See Morgan 2001). The point is that if activities with more inherent meaning were emphasized, it would be easier for people to incorporate them into their routines. Gardening, walking to do an errand, and cycling to work have more inherent meaning than pedaling a stationary bike to nowhere.

This form of lifestyle intervention consists of public health programs that place their emphasis upon the environmental conditions that encourage or inhibit physical activity, and prescribe the creation of activity-supportive environments. For example, adding well-marked, extensive bike lanes throughout a small city would, according to this model, help to create an environment in which people find it safe and easy to bicycle to work or school. Similarly, educational programs that encourage taking the stairs at work instead of the elevator are designed to increase physical activity for people at work. In contrast are structured interventions, programs designed around structured exercise regimens. These latter interventions use guidelines of exercise frequency, intensity, and duration in order to set performance goals for participants—where intensity is the amount of exertion, duration is the amount of elapsed time spent exercising, and frequency is the number of exercise sessions engaged in over a period of time (Bouchard and Shephard 1994). In this type of intervention, public health researchers or practitioners take a direct role in getting people to participate in structured activities such as aerobics dance classes.

Lifestyle interventions have been shown to be as effective, and in some cases more effective, than structured interventions in overcoming the adoption and adherence hurdles. Lifestyle interventions can yield positive and long-term effects, in terms of increasing the levels of moderately intense physical activity and in reducing the levels of sedentariness within studied groups (Dunn et al. 1998). Those who are sedentary or mostly inactive are more likely to be more responsive to lifestyle interventions that encourage the adoption of moderately intense, inexpensive, and convenient forms of physical activity (Shephard 1997). Moderate activities of shorter duration may allow people to more readily fit physical activity into their daily schedule and habit patterns. Moreover, the lower intensity threshold allows sedentary people to start engaging in the activity without fear of the physical pain that accompanies vigorous exercise. Moderate physical activities also typically require less in the way of specialized equipment and/or access to specialized facilities, and may generate less apprehension for the beginner with respect to the social embarrassment that may accompany working out at a fitness facility. In contrast, vigorous activities in structured settings present a number of barriers: they simply may be too difficult, time-consuming, or embarrassing for many people, especially for people who are elderly, overweight/obese, or out of shape due to a prolonged sedentary lifestyle. In addition, people may be physically unable or mentally unprepared to participate in vigorous activities like jogging or aerobics over the long term.

An example of the effectiveness of lifestyle interventions is provided by a study published in the *Journal of the American Medical Association*. A group of researchers tracked how well two different interventions did at improving levels of physical activity, cardiorespiratory fitness, and cardiovascular disease risk factors amongst 235 adults. The study consisted of six months of direct interventions wherein the researchers monitored and encouraged participation; eighteen months of maintenance intervention (where the intervention was less frequent and intense) followed. One group was assigned to a lifestyle intervention program wherein participants were simply encouraged to engage in moderate physical activities; the main components of this intervention focused on education. The other group was placed in a highly structured exercise program that consisted of enrolling participants in a health club. Results from the six months of direct intervention showed that the lifestyle physical activity intervention was as effective in increasing physical activity as the structured program. During the eighteen-month follow-up, the authors found that both groups continued to enjoy significant and comparable improvements in physical activity levels, cardiorespiratory fitness, blood pressure, and percentage of body fat (Dunn et al. 1999). Other studies have shown similar results, with lifestyle interventions performing as well as structured interventions in lowering weight, systolic blood pressure, and serum lipid and lipoprotein levels (Andersen et al. 1999). Once such activities are begun, participants are more likely to continue and to obtain long-term improvements in levels of physical activity (Dunn, Andersen, and Jakicic 1998). For these reasons, less strenuous forms of exercise may be more effective in inducing long-term changes in the behavior of sedentary adults (Owen and Bauman 1992).

Walking and bicycling are important in this context because they are two types of moderately intense physical activity that can be incorporated easily into daily routines in the built environment. Walking improves cardiovascular capacity, bodily endurance, lower body muscular strength and flexibility, posture, enhances metabolism of lipoproteins and insulin/glucose dynamics, and may increase bone strength (Morris and Hardman 1997). Walking may also help to manage arthritis—one study reported that regular walking reduces pain and improves function in people with knee arthritis (Kovar et al. 1992). In fact walking is a core component of many arthritis treatments programs. Walking is the most readily available form of physical activity in the world, as most people can and do engage in it every day, and thus is the easiest form of physical activity to undertake. As a result, walking is ideal as a start-up activity for the sedentary, the overweight/obese, and the elderly, because of its simplicity and low threshold of activity (Morris and Hardman 1997; Shephard 1997).

As with walking, cycling's independent effects on health continue to accumulate. In Europe, where cycling rates are much higher than in the U.S., there is a growing body of research suggesting that cycling for transportation or recreation can provide significant health benefits. For example, a number of studies have reported a lower risk of death for those who are active cyclists (for recreation or transportation) compared with those who are not (Andersen et al. 1999; Oja, Vuori, and Paronen 1998; Vuori, Oja, and Paronen 1994; Hillman 1992). It is also less stressful on joints and bones than is walking. Although cycling is slightly less accessible than walking (cycling requires some equipment, obviously, and also requires more balance and coordination than walking), it is an activity that most of the population can engage in if they so choose. The number of bicycles in the United States, at 100 million or more, alone testifies to the viability and affordability of this form of physical activity.

Conclusion

A consensus is developing within public health circles that lifestyles are key to understanding chronic disease patterns in the general population, leading to calls for more research into the underlying behavioral trends and patterns that produce chronic diseases and conditions. The dramatically increasing levels of overweight and obesity in the United States have also served to point many in the public health community toward understanding how poor dietary and physical activity patterns contribute to these problems. As this chapter has shown, there is increasing evidence suggesting that nonstructured forms of exercise can be a critical component in improving Americans' overall health. This perspective derives additional force from the fact that so many people get very little exercise, and even though most say they would like to be more active, they seem to have a hard time increasing the amount of activity they get. Because such a large percentage of the population is sedentary or only active occasionally, and because more health risks accrue to people within this category than for those who are more frequent exercisers, public health researchers repeatedly stress the need to activate sedentary individuals. The rationale is threefold: moderate forms of exercise such as walking can actually be performed by beginning exercisers, whereas more strenuous forms of exercise such as aerobic dance may be too difficult; moderate exercise can be more easily worked into a person's daily routines, becoming a part of one's lifestyle and thus requiring no long-term commitment to a structured exercise program at a facility; and adherence rates to exercise programs consisting of moderate and purposeful exercise may be higher than those involving more strenuous forms.

CHAPTER FOUR

Physical Activity

TYPES AND PATTERNS

> Given the health benefits of regular physical activity, we have to wonder
> why two out of three Americans are continuing to risk their health and
> the quality of their lives by remaining sedentary.
>
> U.S. DEPARTMENT OF HEALTH AND HUMAN SERVICES,
> *Promoting Physical Activity: A Guide for Community Action* (1999)

There are many different types of physical activity, and each has different attributes, qualities, and purposes, which collectively determine how easy or difficult it is to adopt and adhere to each type. Physical activity can be either recreational or utilitarian in nature, demand either a moderate or a vigorous amount of exertion from the participant, and require varying amounts of leisure time, financial resources, and equipment. This chapter makes the case that, all other things being equal, activities that have a lower exertion threshold, require little equipment or financial resources, do not take much time from other activities, and have some practical purpose have distinct advantages over other types. We argue that walking and bicycling are advantaged in this respect, in particular the fact that they are moderately intense, impose relatively few barriers on those wishing to begin participation in them, and, perhaps most importantly, can be done by a person while he or she is performing some other useful task. Unfortunately, the levels of walking and bicycling for utilitarian purposes in the United States are very low. In many wealthy countries in other parts of the world, walking and bicycling are much more common, suggesting that the strikingly low levels of nonmotorized travel in the United States may be the result of environmental and other factors that are unique to this country.

The Evaluation of Physical Activity Types

There are a very large number of specific types of physical activity—running, weight lifting, racquetball, mountain climbing, bicycling, tennis, badminton, aerobics, and so on. Despite the variation in physical activity types, however, it is possible to place each within a systematic typology. In chapter 3 we discussed a few dimensions along which physical activity types can be examined, for instance, the exertion level needed to participate in an activity. As was claimed, physical activity does not have to be high in exertion in order to generate health benefits. In this section, two additional categories are introduced and discussed, one that addresses the purpose of an activity and the other the obstacles to participating in an activity.

RECREATIONAL VERSUS UTILITARIAN ACTIVITY

As the name implies, recreational forms of exercise are those undertaken for discretionary reasons on someone's leisure time. When most people think about physical activity, they are usually thinking about these forms of exercise. Examples include a wide array of familiar activities: jogging, weight lifting, hiking, basketball, soccer, and so on. In contrast, utilitarian exercise consists of those physical activities that are undertaken in order to accomplish another purpose. The classic example is walking or bicycling to work, school, or the store. In this example, the physical activity—walking or bicycling—is a by-product of achieving some other goal that the person has in mind. While a person has perhaps chosen to walk or bicycle, as opposed to driving, the fulfillment of some other objective is the primary purpose of the exercise.

The built environment influences both types of physical activity. Because recreational exercise occurs in or on parks, playgrounds, baseball diamonds, basketball courts, and biking trails, to name just a few places, the spatial allocation of these facilities is important. An intuitive hypothesis is that the proximity of such facilities to one's residence or workplace has an independent influence on a person's ability and desire to engage in recreational exercise. In this case, intuition appears to be on the mark. In 2001, the Task Force on Community Preventive Services, an independent team of public health schol-

ars, conducted a rigorous and systematic review of community-based interventions designed to promote physical activity. Based upon this review, the
Task Force recommended interventions that serve to "create or enhance
access to places for physical activity," by which they meant trails, parks, and
other recreational facilities in the built environment (CDC 2001a). A common lament about conventional suburban development is that few subdivisions are built with recreational facilities such as sports fields, parks, and
playgrounds contained within them (conversely, however, some private
developments, usually in the form of gated communities, offer private exercise facilities). As state and local governments struggle to build enough parks
and other recreational facilities to keep up with the frenzied pace of suburban development, one result is an increase in the amount of distance one has
to travel to reach such a facility. To illustrate, figure 4-1 provides some results
of an analysis of regional travel data from Seattle collected in 1996. The figure shows that people in the oldest areas of Seattle traveled fewer miles in
order to reach recreational destinations than those who lived in the newest
developments.[1] This evidence suggests that older, more traditional neighborhoods possess attributes that reduce the need for long trips to and from
recreational destinations, while newer neighborhoods do not possess these
attributes. Older neighborhoods, moreover, typically possess amenities that
make certain types of physical activity, including recreational and utilitarian
walking and bicycling, more attractive and desirable.[2]

The built environment's influence on recreational exercise is not limited
to how close facilities such as parks are to residential areas. Even if a facility
is proximate to homes or offices, it may be underutilized because it is of low
quality, is perceived as an unsafe place, or is difficult to reach. Many city parks
have facilities that are in poor condition. Some parks are also seen as unsafe,
viewed as places where drugs are dealt and crimes are committed. Parks and
other recreational facilities may be difficult to reach using certain types of
transportation. Even if a facility is near one's residence, if street crossings near
the facility are hazardous or if there are few sidewalks along the street leading to the facility, a person may not be able to safely reach the facility on foot
or by bicycle. For vulnerable groups such as children, the elderly, and low-
income people, this consideration may have greater relevance simply because
members of these groups have a more difficult time getting to the facility.

While recreational physical activity is undertaken for its own sake and

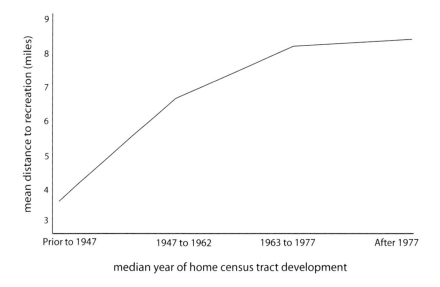

FIGURE 4-1. Average distance to travel from home to recreational destinations, Seattle area, 1996. Source: 1996 Puget Sound Transportation Panel survey.

during one's leisure time, utilitarian forms of physical activity are those that are worked into one's daily habits. Utilitarian physical activity has the potential to be more important than recreational exercise precisely because it is integrated into other activities. A major reason is the amount of discretionary or leisure time that people have available to them. Finding the time to engage in recreational exercise to meet the recommended levels of moderate activity, thirty minutes or more on most or all days of the week, is challenging for people if they rely solely on recreational physical activity. Other personal factors, including fatigue and lack of motivation, also constrain people's ability to get enough recreational exercise. In the case of the majority of Americans who do not get enough exercise to meet public health guidelines, utilitarian physical activity may very well be the only type of physical activity that people who face these constraints could get on a daily basis, were the built environment constructed in such a way as to allow for it.

PERSONAL VERSUS ENVIRONMENTAL BARRIERS TO PHYSICAL ACTIVITY

Different types of recreational and utilitarian physical activity vary with respect to who can participate in the activity, when it can be done, and where facilities exist for the activity to be performed. The advantages and disadvantages of each can be categorized and described through the concept of barriers to exercise. Barriers are obstacles that inhibit or prevent one's ability to adopt and, once begun, to adhere to an activity over time. There are two types of barriers, personal and environmental. Personal barriers include such things as one's level of motivation, physical capabilities, amount of leisure time available, financial resources, and the extent of family, work, and household obligations. Environmental barriers are obstacles that are imposed by the built environment and, occasionally, the natural environment (e.g., the weather). These barriers include the availability of facilities for different types of physical activity, the distance between home and such facilities or other destinations, and the perceived quality and safety of the environment in which one wishes to participate in a certain activity.

The most commonly reported personal barrier is a lack of time for exercise. Other frequently cited personal barriers include a physical inability to exercise (perceived or real), a lack of motivation, a lack of social support for exercise, fatigue, childcare responsibilities, and a lack of health knowledge (Booth et al. 1997; Myers and Roth 1997; Sallis et al. 1986). Environmental barriers include all of those things in the built environment that impede physical activity; an example would be the absence of bike lanes on roads. Unfortunately, while personal barriers have enjoyed a good deal of attention, public health research has not been as comprehensive in examining the effects of environmental barriers on physical activity. Models of individual behavioral change have acknowledged the importance of social psychology and the social environment for some time, but few public health models have explicitly specified the role of the physical environment in influencing public health (Sallis and Owen 1990). Nonetheless, in recent years there have been increasing calls by some public health researchers to recognize the importance of the built environment (see, e.g., Powell, Bricker, and Blair 2002). There is some understanding that policies aimed at reducing environmental barriers may have the potential to increase physical activity more than policies aimed at influencing individual behavior. This argument has gotten much of its force from the general failure of attempts to change individual behavior in the United States through the types of structured approaches that were reviewed in the last chapter. It is unreasonable, some have argued, to expect people to change their behaviors when the environment discourages such changes (Schmid, Pratt, and Howze 1995).

Additional impetus has also come from a few public health studies that have worked environmental barriers into their research designs. One, conducted by researchers at the School of Public Health at Saint Louis University (Brownson et al. 2001), found from survey data that having a supportive environment near one's home (lots of sidewalks, low traffic levels, etc.) was associated with greater levels of physical activity. This finding led the authors to call for integrating environmental strategies, which aim to alter or control the physical environments in which people live, into public health interventions so as to encourage or discourage certain patterns of behavior. Similarly, the results from an older study conducted in San Diego (Linenger, Chesson, and Nice 1991) examined changes in physical fitness levels amongst personnel at a military base. The researchers changed the environment at the base (by constructing bicycle paths, extending hours at recreation facilities, installing new exercise equipment at the station's gym, organizing running and cycling clubs, creating institutional support and rewards for physical activity, and changing the menus at food establishments). The results of the study found significantly greater levels of physical fitness at the experimental community after the intervention occurred. While this study contained elements of both types of interventions, lifestyle and structured, the researchers believed that their intervention allowed people to take advantage of the environmental changes that were offered to them.

Research into environmental interventions has been hampered by a lack of empirically grounded models of how the environment influences physical activity. Public health researchers have been attempting to fill the void through the creation of conceptual models that tie behavior to the built environment. An example is provided in figure 4-2, created by three public health researchers: James Sallis, Adrian Bauman, and Michael Pratt. Their model focused on the importance of those settings, facilities, and programs that they believed would encourage physical activity. According to their theoretical structure, public policies influence physical activity levels, either directly as in the case of educational programs or indirectly through the ways that they structure the environments in which people live, play, and work (Sallis, Bauman, and Pratt 1998).

Physical Activity Types: A Summary Comparison

Table 4-1 provides an assessment of some examples of physical activity. In the table, each is evaluated along four dimensions. First, each type is given a rating corresponding with the level of exertion required to perform the activity, from moderate to vigorous exertion. Second, each is categorized according to its purpose, whether it is recreational or utilitarian in nature. Third, each is given a rating based upon the number of barriers that a person needs to overcome in order to participate. Here, the barriers include whether the activity requires a high skill threshold level (e.g., the activity requires substantial agility, skill, or coordination), specialized equipment and facilities, leisure time, and other participants. Finally, each type of physical activity is given a summary rating. This takes into consideration the level of exertion required, the purpose of the activity, and the types of personal and environmental barriers to participating in the activity. The summary rating indicates how difficult it is to adopt each type of physical activity and, once adopted, how difficult it is to adhere to the activity over the long term.

The activities listed include high intensity team sports (soccer, basketball), individual sports (tennis, golf, racquetball), standard types of individual exercise (jogging, rowing machine, lap swimming), and walking and bicycling. This table does not contain all types of physical activity, of course, nor does it contain a full listing of all possible barriers, especially the environmental barriers, that people may face when making a decision to undertake the activity. Admittedly, the description and evaluation of each activity listed in table 4-1 is somewhat subjective, although the specified exertion level for each type of activity is in accordance with the categorization schemes of public health agencies (see table for further information). Nonetheless, the purpose of the table is illustrative: to describe the unique attributes of each type

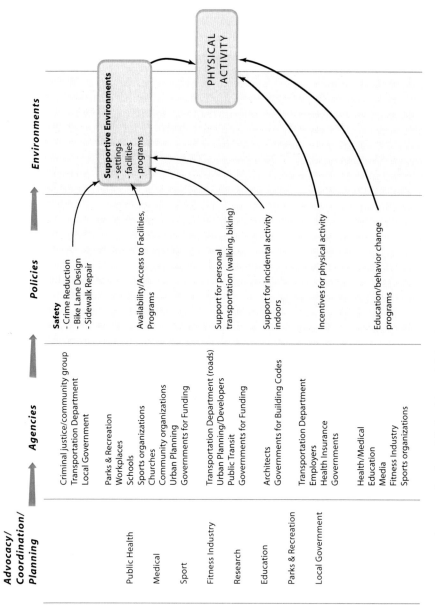

FIGURE 4-2. An example of a public health model that focuses on the environmental bases of physical activity. Source: Reprinted by permission of Elsevier Science from "Environmental and policy interventions to promote physical activity," James Sallis, Adrian Bauman and Michael Pratt, *American Journal of Preventive Medicine*, Vol. 15 No. 4, pp. 379–97. Copyright 1998 by *American Journal of Preventive Medicine*.

of physical activity and to suggest how easily or difficult each type is adopted and adhered to over time.

Each activity possesses a unique combination of attributes in terms of exertion level, purpose, and barriers to adoption and adherence. According to the table, for instance, golf requires a moderate amount of exertion (note that the only type of golf considered here is one where the player walks, carrying or wheeling a bag; playing golf while riding in a cart does not require a moderate amount of exertion). The purpose of golf is strictly recreational (not counting, of course, so-called business golf outings). Golf has two primary barriers. Participants need specialized equipment such as clubs and golf balls, which are usually expensive. Just as importantly, they need a place to play—a golf course—which requires the payment of fees for its use. For these reasons, in table 4-1 golf is given a middle rating in terms of the difficulty the average person would have in taking up golf and sticking to it over the long term. Golf requires lots of leisure time and a lot of money, two commodities that many people do not have. It may be objected that the popularity of golf provides evidence against this thesis, that because so many people play golf there must be few difficulties in getting people to adopt and adhere to this activity. While it is true that millions of people play golf, much of the time golfers are playing while riding in motorized carts, which do not require nearly the same level of exertion as walking a course. Moreover, golf is still a pastime that entire segments of the population are excluded from playing. For example, low-income people have few discretionary resources and therefore find it more difficult to play such a resource-intensive sport.

The same logic has been applied to all of the activities in the table. The team and individual sports require high exertion, are recreational activities, and have relatively high personal barriers to participation (in terms of leisure time, equipment, cost, need for a specialized facility, and other attributes). For the majority of the population that is completely sedentary or irregularly active, these more vigorous forms of physical activity will be difficult to adopt because of the high physical exertion required. Once adopted, long-term adherence will be difficult because of the need for sufficient leisure time, access to specialized facilities, and, in some cases, for the conditions under which the activity must be done, for example as in team sports where other players are required.

TABLE 4-1
Types of physical activity: Analysis and evaluation

Type of Activity	Exertion level*		Activity purpose		Barriers to participation				Level of difficulty for adoption and adherence		
	Moderate	Vigorous	Utilitarian	Recreational	High physical threshold	Equipment/ facilities needed	Leisure time required	Other participants required	Low	Mid	High
Walking	x		x	x					x		
Bicycling	x	x	x	x					x	x	
Jogging		x		x	x		x				x
Rowing machine		x		x	x	x	x				x
Singles tennis		x		x	x	x	x	x			x
Golf (walking)	x			x		x	x			x	
Lap swimming		x		x	x	x	x				x
Raquetball or squash		x		x	x	x	x	x			x
High intensity team sports		x		x	x	x	x	x			x

*Definition and classification of exertion levels as provided by U.S. Department of Health and Human Services et al. (1999), Table 2.1. Moderate physical activity defined as activity that produces 3.0 to 6.0 METs, with vigorous activity producing greater than 6.0 METs. MET = "metabolic equivalent," a ratio of exercise metabolic rate to resting metabolic rate. One MET is the energy expended while sitting; for an adult this translates into approximately 3.5 ml of oxygen uptake per kilogram of body weight per minute.

The Case for Walking and Bicycling

Table 4-1 also provides the basis for claiming that walking and bicycling are the two types of physical activity that are the easiest to adopt and adhere to over the long term—they are the only types of physical activity that warrant a "low" summary rating. Why do we believe that these two types of activity should appeal to the broadest set of people? First, the level of exertion *required* to participate in each is low. Bicycling is given both a moderate and a vigorous assessment because bicycling can take many forms, ranging from an easy ride around the block to road and mountain bike racing, which are very strenuous sports, to long-distance touring. Second, while both walking and bicycling are common forms of recreational physical activity, they also can be utilitarian forms of physical activity, since both are practical means of transport to school, work, or shopping. Third, these forms of activity impose few barriers on participants. Neither requires significant time investment, financial resources, or facilities. Even the need for a bicycle is a relatively low barrier, as used and even new entry-level bicycles can be very inexpensive.

All of these qualities add up to a summary rating of low in terms of difficulty in adoption and adherence. Again, bicycling is given a rating from low to high, due to the many different types of bicycling that can be performed. Bicycle racing, for example, is very difficult and requires a sustained commitment to vigorous exercise. Yet for the majority, both bicycling and walking are simple forms of exercise. For those who are elderly, infirm, overweight or obese, or sedentary, walking and bicycling are appealing because the exertion threshold to participate is much lower than for vigorous activities. For those with few material resources, these activities can be done with little or no money. For those who do not have much leisure time, the fact that walking and bicycling can be utilitarian activities provides them with a unique advantage, giving them perhaps the greatest potential single advantage over all other forms of physical activity.

WALKING AND BICYCLING: PATTERNS AND TRENDS
IN THE UNITED STATES AND ABROAD

It is not surprising that the automobile dominates intra-city travel in the United States. According to the U.S. Department of Transportation's

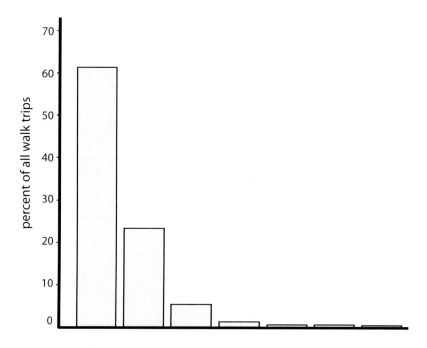

FIGURE 4-3. Walk trip distances, Seattle area, 1996. Source: 1996 Puget Sound Transportation Panel survey.

Nationwide Personal Transportation System (NPTS), travel by private vehicle accounts for 86 percent of all person trips and 91 percent of all person miles, while walking accounts for only 5 percent of trips and less than 1 percent of miles.[3] For work travel, the figures are even more dominated by the auto. Ninety-one percent of commute trips are by car, with walking accounting for only 2 percent of all work trips. Nonwork trips for purposes such as shopping, entertainment, or recreation accounted for 82.7 percent of all trips (Federal Highway Administration [FHWA] 1997). Moreover, trend data reveal that Americans are using the single-occupant vehicle for an increasing percentage of all trips and for greater distances (Hu and Young 1999).

Data from the NPTS show that there are about 56 million walk trips and 9 million bicycle trips in the U.S. each day. Most of these appear to be for nonutilitarian purposes, with people responding to survey questionnaires that personal and social reasons account for the majority.[4] As one can expect, the distance traveled in the average walk or bike trip is a limiting factor in the

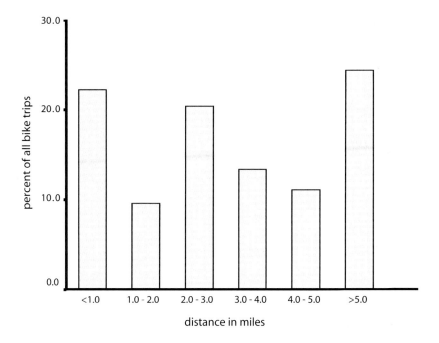

FIGURE 4-4. Bicycle trip distances, Seattle area, 1996. Source: 1996 Puget Sound Transportation Panel survey.

usefulness of these modes for meeting utilitarian needs. Most walking trips that are reported in the NPTS are less than one kilometer (two-thirds of a mile), with a majority of bicycling trips between one and eight kilometers (about five miles) (Antonakos 1995). The short nature of nonmotorized trips has been confirmed across different studies in the American context (for example, see the data from the Seattle region contained in figures 4-3 and 4-4). However, there is some cross-national and local evidence to suggest that the average nonmotorized trip length can be significantly longer, depending on the context of the built environment and the behavior of other transportation system users. For example, in the Netherlands, bicycling trips are often much longer than the American average, reflecting the extent to which bicycling is a safe and acceptable means of practical transportation in that country.

Studies yield different findings regarding the demographics of nonmotorized travel. A review conducted by the Federal Highway Administration (FHWA 1994) showed that males cycle more than females, and the young more than the old, with some indication that cycling is most popular for those in their mid-twenties. While most bicyclists ride for recreation or exercise, a small percentage commutes by bicycle. There is some evidence to suggest that serious bicyclists are more affluent than average. Two surveys conducted in the 1990s of bicycle commuters and avid cyclists in Seattle provide support for this position. Data from the survey of avid cyclists (Moritz 1998) revealed that the average respondent was a forty-eight-year-old male professional with a college degree who reported a household income greater than $60,000 per year. The study of bicycle commuters (Moritz 1997) revealed similar findings. The average respondent was a thirty-nine-year-old male professional with a household income greater than $45,000 per year.[5]

Other studies have found that nonmotorists tend to be younger, less educated, and poorer, are more likely to be unemployed or live in urbanized areas, and are less likely to have a driver's license or live in a household with a motor vehicle (Antonakos 1995). The split between male and female nonmotorists is about even. Households with children may make as many as two to three times as many nonmotorized trips as households with no children (Niemeier and Rutherford 1994).

We should pause to note that the amount of research that has been done on nonmotorized travel is significantly less than that for motorized travel. Part of the reason stems from inadequate data or incomplete data collection by public agencies. Nonmotorists are seldom treated on the same level as motorists by those agencies that conduct travel surveys (Wigan 1995). When survey data is gathered in a rigorous and exhaustive fashion, bicycling and walking are often lumped together under the heading of nonmotorized transportation. This is problematic because walking and bicycling differ substantially in terms of the speed at which one moves while engaging in each type of activity, by the facilities and equipment required for each, by the age and demographic profile of the typical user, and by other important issues. Despite all of these problems, however, there are some reliable sources of data on walking and biking at the national level and there have been many studies of pedestrians and bicyclists conducted at the local level.

A safe assumption to make about American attitudes regarding transportation is that people have a preference for travel by the automobile. This, of course, is reflective of the dominance of the automobile in American life, a fact that perhaps leads many to believe that given the choice to drive or use any other means of transport, most people would naturally choose to drive. Yet statistics from some other wealthy industrialized countries show that automobile travel is not nearly as dominant as in the United States. While the car is a very important mode of transportation, other travel modes, including walking and bicycling, enjoy both higher status and higher usage around the world. Data gathered by John Pucher and Christian Lefevre, two transportation researchers who specialize in nonmotorized forms of transportation, reveal that the modal "share" (the breakdown, in percentage terms, of travel by each type of transportation, or mode) differs substantially across wealthy industrial countries (table 4-2). The share of all urban trips taken by car varies from as low as 25 percent in Sweden to a high of 84 percent in the United States, with an average of 52 percent for all of the European and North American countries shown in the table.[6] Bicycling and walking rates are considerably higher in Europe than in the U.S. and Canada, with the United States also ranking last in public transit usage. In several countries, car usage is only slightly above or even slightly below other transportation modes. In Sweden, for example, 39 percent of all trips are made on foot compared to 38 percent by car. When combined, bicycling and walking exceeds or nearly equals that for the automobile in Austria, Denmark, Italy, the Netherlands, Sweden, and Switzerland. At the opposite end of the spectrum are Canada, the United Kingdom, and the United States (Pucher and Lefevre 1996). National statistics from Europe are complemented by very high nonmotorized trip rates at the city level in Europe as well. In Bern, for example, a quarter of all trips are on foot and over 10 percent are by bicycle (Haefeli 2001). In Helsinki, walking trips account for 16 percent of all trips, with bicycling trips at 9 percent and transit at 30 percent. In Utrecht, an astonishing 40 percent of all trips to the downtown are made by bicycle, with another 40 percent by transit (Beatley 2000). Finally, there is some evidence to suggest that nonmotorized travel is not only more frequent in Europe but that the average nonmotorized trip distance may be longer than in the United States. In the Netherlands, bicycling accounted for 24 percent of all trips between 5 and 7.5 kilometers and 11 percent of all trips between 10 and 15 kilometers (Pucher and Lefevre 1996).

It would be inaccurate to imply that automobiles are an unimportant mode of travel in Europe. On the contrary, automobile ownership and use has grown dramatically in Europe, as it has in the United States, over the postwar

TABLE 4-2
Modal split by country (as percentage of total trips) in urban areas, 1990
(or latest available year)

Country	Car	Public transport	Bicycling	Walking
Austria	39	13	9	31
Canada	74	14	1	10
Denmark	42	14	20	21
France	54	12	4	30
Germany	52	11	10	27
Italy*	25	21	54	
Netherlands	44	8	27	19
Norway*	68	7	25	
Sweden	36	11	10	39
Switzerland	38	20	10	29
UK**	62	14	8	12
USA	84	3	1	9
Average***	52	12	10	23

*Statistics for bicycling and walking as separate modes are not available.
**England and Wales.
***Rounded figures.
Means for Bicycling category and Walking category do not include Italy and Norway.
SOURCE: John Pucher and Christian Lefevre, *The Urban Transport Crisis in Europe and North America*, 1996, London: Macmillan Press. Reproduced with permission of Palgrave Macmillan. Data primarily from national transport ministries.

period. European countries have long faced similar difficulties with respect to the automobile's impact on urban form and life. There is also a great deal of variation in Europe in the rates at which people use alternative modes of travel, both spatially (within individual cities as well as across countries) and demographically (wealthy Europeans compared to poorer ones). However, it remains true that in many parts of Europe, transit and nonmotorized modes are enormously popular means of transportation, far more popular than in the United States.

What, then, explains the continuing differences between the United States and many parts of Europe? Certainly, the high taxes levied on fuel in Europe are important, acting as a suppressant on the demand for driving. However, at least some of the explanation lies in urban form issues. To start with, the transportation infrastructure is very different. Most European cities have transit systems that are much better than all but a very small number of systems in the United States, allowing a person to move around a city without the use of a car. Because walking and, depending on the transit system's design, bicycling are natural complements of transit (see chapter 7), the prospects for nonmotorized travel are greatly heightened by efficient and ubiquitous transit systems. In contrast to the United States, Europeans invest heavily in rail and bus transit systems in the belief that the investment of public funds in transit infrastructure has positive social and environmental utility that outweighs the fiscal burden. Conversely, public policies are often crafted in order to increase the monetary cost of owning and operating a car and to impose other constraints on automobile use so as to improve the competitive position of transit and nonmotorized modes; such policies are widespread in Switzerland, Germany, the Netherlands, and the Nordic countries (Vuchic 1999). Another obvious point has to do with the ways that European cities are built. There, public policies support and often require private development to conform to an urban development model that stresses high densities of population (relative to the United States) and a mix of land uses (where stores and offices, for example, are near housing). Compact urban development makes both transit and nonmotorized modes of transportation viable because the distances between destinations are short and because people are concentrated in a smaller area.

There are numerous examples of how such policies improve nonmotorized travel and transit while stemming the growth in auto based travel. John Pucher reports that Freiburg, a small city located in southwestern Germany, has for decades had innovative policies designed to increase travel by these modes while decreasing auto use. The city has created a large pedestrian zone, hundreds of kilometers of bike lanes and paths, pedestrian- and bicyclist-friendly traffic regulations, has installed thousands of bike racks, and has eliminated much of the free on-street parking in the city center. Additionally, the city has worked to reduce the roadway capacity for automobiles within the city core, by narrowing residential streets, and emplacing obstacles to vehicle movement on residential streets such as street tree plantings, and other devices. Simultaneously, the city has worked to improve the accessibility to these areas by the other three modes: transit, walking, and bicycling. The result is that these modes combine for some 64 percent of all trips in Freiburg, with the car accounting for only 36 percent (Pucher 1998; Pucher and Clorer 1992). While Freiburg and other progressive cities are more aggressive in implementing these strategies than other German cities, similar tools are widely used in Germany. Large pedestrian zones, for example, are commonplace, the result of deliberate decisions by towns and cities in the last few decades to redesign core urban areas, especially historic districts, around the pedestrian. Despite the well-known love affair that many Germans have with the automobile, between 1966 and 1986, German municipalities managed to increase the number of such zones from 63 to around 800 for the whole of the former West Germany (Monheim 1986).

These comparative statistics underscore how the built environment plays a critical role in shaping the travel options that a person has. Walking and bicycling are much more convenient and enjoyable in European cities because these cities have been designed to make them that way. They are also, not coincidentally, safer. It is much more dangerous to walk or bicycle in the United States than in the Netherlands and Germany. Fatality rates for pedestrians are ten times higher than in either of these two countries (on a per-kilometer basis), while those for bicyclists are four times higher (Pucher and Dijkstra 2000; Pucher 2001).

Such data on safety only describes objective conditions. Most Americans are fully aware that their cities are unsafe, unpleasant, and impractical for walking and bicycling and shift their behavior accordingly. Responses to surveys in places with low rates of walking and bicycling generally show that people are very concerned about poor environmental conditions and change their behavior as a result (CDC 1999b; Go for Green/Environics 1998). Seemingly objective concepts as safety and distance are really both subjective and objective phenomena, and the two interact to influence how willing people are to walk or bicycle (table 4-3). Distance between destinations is, of course, measurable, but a person's perception of distance is also influenced by other factors as well, such as the quality of the route in between destinations.

WALKING AND BICYCLING: LATENT DEMAND

Put simply, the built environment has been constructed in a way that prohibits most travel by any means other than the car. Some evidence exists to support the view that there is a gap between how people currently travel and how they wish they could travel. Surveys about how people would like to travel reveal that walking and bicycling would be more popular if safe and accessible transportation networks for these alternatives were available. For example, in 1995 Rodale Press, a Pennsylvania research and publishing firm, commissioned a nationwide survey of 1,000 adults that focused on the availability of facilities for walking and bicycling. While only 3 percent of respondents said that they walked as their primary means of travel, 7 percent of

TABLE 4-3
Factors influencing walking and bicycling

Personal and subjective factors	Environmental factors
Distance	Distance
Traffic safety	Traffic safety
Convenience	Weather
Cost	Topography
Valuation of time	*Infrastructure:*
Valuation of exercise	• Pedestrian/bike facilities, traffic conditions
Physical condition	
Habits	• Access and likage of pedestrian/bicycle
	facilities to desireable destinations
Attitude and values	
Peer group acceptance	• Existence of competitive transportation alternatives

SOURCE: Federal Highway Administration 1994.

respondents said that they would most prefer to walk, assuming that good facilities for walking existed. The figures were similar for bicycling: only 2 percent said they bicycled as their primary means of travel, but 6 percent said that they would most prefer to bicycle as their primary means of travel if good facilities existed. In contrast, while 76 percent of the respondents said that driving alone was their primary means of travel, only 56 percent said that they would most prefer to drive as their primary means of travel (Rodale Press 1995). In Canada, which has transportation patterns not too dissimilar to those in the United States, a 1998 national survey of 1,500 adults also generated evidence that Canadians desire more opportunities for biking and walking. Eight in ten respondents said that they would like to walk more than they already do, while two out of three stated that they would ideally like to bicycle more. Of the survey respondents, 70 percent indicated that they would cycle to work if there were dedicated bike lanes that would allow for travel to work within thirty minutes (Go for Green/Environics 1998).

The constraints imposed by the contemporary built environment have been a driving force behind New Urbanism, the term for a loose coalition of architects and planners who believe in the virtues of traditional neighborhood design. Its advocates claim that the design elements found in traditional neighborhoods (usually defined as having been built prior to World War II) offer a more pleasant, efficient, and livable environment for their residents than that offered by the contemporary suburb. New Urbanism is built upon the idea that many Americans are tired of conventional suburban development and are willing to pay for an alternative. Its chief proponents routinely cite a mismatch between the typical suburban environment and the desires that people have to live in human-scaled and walkable places.[7] Peter Calthorpe, one of New Urbanism's leading figures, wrote in his landmark 1993 book *The Next American Metropolis,* "pedestrians are the catalyst which makes the essential qualities of communities meaningful. . . . Their absence in our thinking and planning is a fundamental source of failure in our new developments" (Calthorpe 1993, 17). Clearly, these architects believe that a substantial portion of the home-buying public wants neighborhoods that are scaled more to the nonmotorist and less to the automobile. This view has been bolstered by impressionistic evidence as well as more rigorous survey data showing that people are not fully satisfied with the range of housing and neighborhood choices available to them (e.g., Myers and Gearin 2002). New Urbanists such as Calthorpe, Andres Duany, and others have been more than willing to put these ideas to the test: the developments that both men have been involved in, such as the now-famous Seaside, Florida, and Laguna West, California, communities, have a significant pedestrian orientation. It must be said, however, that this movement is not without its critics. New Urbanism has been critiqued as being little more than a cover for rebuilding suburbia so that the wealthy can live in pedestrian-oriented enclaves at the urban fringe. There is merit in this critique, as New Urban developments have tended to be built on the urban fringe and, in many cases, are places where only the wealthy can afford to live. However, the point here is not whether New Urbanism is the architectural paradigm that should supplant conventional development. Rather, it is that New Urbanism's success demonstrates that there is a demand for more pedestrian-oriented spaces in the United States.

Conclusion

Physical activity is a diverse phenomenon. Each type varies along several dimensions, including the level of exertion required (moderately to vigorously intense), its purpose (recreational or utilitarian), the amount of leisure time required, and the number and type of barriers that face the potential participant. Each type of physical activity therefore possesses advantages and disadvantages: it can be easy or difficult, require a good deal of time or relatively little time, and so forth. Among the many different types of activities that can be engaged in within the built environment, walking and bicycling possess a number of advantages that make them more likely to be adopted and maintained over the long term; these include such things as the low activity thresholds needed and the low financial resources required to begin these activities. The potential for utilitarian walking and bicycling may be much higher than that for recreational walking and bicycling because utilitarian forms can be worked more easily into daily living patterns.

A variety of subjective and objective barriers inhibit walking and bicycling. Considerations such as time, poor health, and lack of motivation are intertwined with those features of the built environment that make nonmotorized travel difficult, unsafe, inconvenient, or even impossible. Large distances between one's origin and desired destination, for example, are an important barrier. So too are considerations such as traffic safety issues, bad roads for cycling, a lack of sidewalks, and other negative features of the built environment. The decision to walk or bicycle can thus be seen as a function of subjective factors such as perceptions about safety and objective factors such as the state of the built environment and the cost tradeoffs (monetary and temporal) between different modes, such as driving versus transit versus walking or biking.

CHAPTER FIVE

Physical Activity

CHILDREN, THE ELDERLY, AND THE POOR

The automobile has given improved mobility primarily to the middle class, middle aged. But these owner-drivers have not merely gained new mobility through the car; they have also rearranged the physical location patterns of society to suit their own private needs, and unwittingly in the process destroyed and severely limited the mobility and access of all others.

K. H. SCHAEFFER AND ELLIOTT SCLAR,
Access for All: Transportation and Urban Growth (1980)

It is clear by now that physical activity is not a uniform phenomenon. It varies significantly by type, by purpose, and by location of activity as well as by the characteristics of the participant. There are important distinctions between sedentary and active individuals, for example. The population is diverse with respect to other characteristics as well. Many types of recreational physical activity can be, and are, engaged in by a large number of people in their free time. However, only the relatively fit and able-bodied who have sufficient resources—time and money—to engage in these activities can actually do so. Many cannot or will not do so because they are old or infirm, out of shape or lacking in other resources. Differences between advantaged and disadvantaged groups remain even when considering moderate forms of physical activity such as walking and bicycling. Environmental conditions will have divergent effects on different strata within the population.

For groups who enjoy certain personal and financial resources, the built environment places fewer constraints on their behavior and opportunities. For others who do not possess such resources, the story is remarkably different. In the mid-1970s, two social scientists, K. H. Schaeffer and Elliott Sclar, argued that the pattern of decentralized growth in the United States systematically discriminated against members of disadvantaged groups by inhibiting their access to social and economic goods. They argued that environments designed around the automobile, as was the case in the majority of places then as it is now, makes sense only for some portions of the population. Those who can marshal the fewest private resources, where resources are defined in terms of money, physical capabilities, and official license for motorized travel, have the most problems in terms of accessing such goods. They simply have fewer options with respect to travel for utilitarian, recreational, and social purposes. This critique served to highlight the inequities inherent in building cities according to modern principles. The long distances between destinations that are a hallmark of the modern American city not only deprives those who cannot drive, they also make travel by other modes difficult, impractical, and dangerous.

In this chapter we discuss how the built environment affects physical activity patterns among children, the elderly, and the poor. In the case of the elderly, diminished capabilities can prevent or dramatically reduce their ability and desire to engage in physical activity in the built environment. Slower walking speeds, impaired hearing or eyesight, and other problems often convince the elderly that their best option is to reduce their exposure to the built environment. For children, their small size and limited experience present obstacles to safe play and movement from destination to destination while outdoors. For the poor, their economic status simply constrains the range of available choices in the built environment, resulting in less frequent, slower, and/or more dangerous travel.

These groups do not define the entire spectrum of vulnerable populations—their inclusion in this chapter is meant to illustrate how society is heterogeneous with respect to physical activity and the built environment. The discussion is not intended to imply that the needs of other groups are unimportant. The physically disabled, for example, is an important group, but the diversity of problems faced by disabled people makes it difficult to generalize about the ways that the built environment systematically constrains their physical activity patterns. Disabilities are very different in type and acuity, for example, ranging from problems involving the senses—eyesight and hearing—to different types of issues involving the limbs, the spinal cord, and other parts of the body. As a result, there is a widely divergent set of solutions with respect to built environment problems for members of this group. In addition, it is difficult to place the needs of the disabled in the context of the physical activity patterns that constitute the bulk of the discussion in this book. Much of this book is concerned with how the built environment influences walking and bicycling, two forms of physical activity that may not be accessible to many of the physically disabled, in particular those with severe disabilities. A final complication involves the fact that physical disabilities cut across all other groups in society, including those discussed in this chapter. Physical disabilities become more common with advancing age, and thus form an important part of the overall health portrait of the elderly.

The three groups chosen for discussion in this chapter are amongst the largest in society, representing a substantial percentage of the American population. Table 5-1, providing statistics from the 2000 Census, shows that children (seventeen years old and younger) constitute about a quarter of the general population, the elderly (sixty-five years old and up) about 12 percent, and the poor 11 percent. It should be noted that the definition of impoverishment that is used by the Census Bureau includes only those people whom the bureau defines as being below the official poverty line established by the federal government. Therefore, the 11 percent figure represents only a fraction of those who might be considered to be "poor" in the United States, as those in income categories that are above the official definition of impoverishment may still be defined as poor or low income.

Children

As was discussed briefly in chapter 3, regular physical activity has many important health benefits for children, including aerobic capacity, weight maintenance, and the psychological benefits that accompany physical fitness as a child or adolescent. In addition to the immediate health benefits of physical activity for children, being active as a child can yield benefits that accrue later in life. Regular physical activity during childhood may help to reduce the chances of suffering from chronic diseases in later years; some chronic diseases, such as heart disease and osteoporosis, have their origins in the earliest decades of life (Sallis and Owen 1999). Moreover, if children are regularly active, there is some expectation a foundation will be established for later phys-

TABLE 5-1.
Percent of U.S. population in vulnerable groups

Group	Population (millions)	Percent of U.S. population
Total U.S. Population (2000)	281.4	100.00
Children (0–17 years)	70.4	25.0
0–5 years	22.7	8.1
6–11 years	24.1	8.6
12–17 years	23.5	8.4
Elderly (65 and over)	35.0	12.4
65-74 years	18.4	6.5
75 and over	16.6	5.9
Impoverished*	31.1	11.1

*The Census Bureau uses money income thresholds to arrive at an official definition of poverty. The poverty threshold varies by household size and composition.
SOURCES: U.S. Bureau of the Census 2001a, 2001b, 2001c.

ical activity patterns, which would have positive health benefits throughout their lifetime (Malina 2001; Telema et al. 1997; Rowland and Freedson 1994).

In recent years, there has been a good deal of concern about the state of children's health in the United States. Much of this has centered on the phenomenon of childhood obesity, which has greatly increased over the last several decades (from 4 to 6 percent during the 1960s to 13 to 14 percent today). Obese children tend to suffer from numerous side effects, running the risk of elevated blood pressures, hypertension, orthopedic abnormalities, sleep disorders, lower pulmonary capacity, emotional problems as the result of peer discrimination, and, in girls, menstrual abnormalities (Strauss 1999). Once a child is classified as overweight or obese, they have a greater chance of remaining in these categories into adulthood; perhaps three-quarters of overweight children go on to be overweight as adults (Freedman et al. 2001).

Such high rates of overweight and obesity point toward systematic linkages between environmental conditions, personal behavior, and body weight. While there is considerable debate over the extent of the role played by genetics in childhood obesity, studies on twins and adopted children have demonstrated that between 20 percent and 50 percent of the variation in body fat are not genetic in origin. The doubling of severe childhood obesity from early 1960 must be partially explained, therefore, by environmental and behavioral factors (Strauss 1999). Past research has documented that eating habits play a significant role in shaping the overweight and obesity trends in children. Another important factor is that children simply are not getting enough physical activity. While children have more time and energy and are therefore more active than adults, data suggests that even among this age group there are worrisome signs that physical inactivity is a large problem. In general terms, children spend much more time engaging in highly sedentary activities such as watching television than they do in active pursuits, a phenomenon that is well-established and shows no signs of abating (Stephens 2002). As they get older, the problem worsens, in particular during the teenage years. Part of the problem stems from biological changes that begin to induce lower levels of physical inactivity, a process that continues throughout life. Data routinely show that rates of physical activity are higher for younger high school students than for older ones. Nationwide in 2001, 72 percent of ninth graders met physical activity guidelines through vigorous activity, while only 56 percent of seniors (twelfth grade) did so. By the time adolescents transition into adulthood, physical inactivity is acute—nearly 40 percent of all high school seniors do not meet health guidelines for physical activity (Grunbaum et al. 2002).[1] Yet while it is true that people become less active with age, external factors are important in determining the rate of decline (Rowland 1999).

CHILDREN AND UTILITARIAN PHYSICAL ACTIVITY

The built environment should be considered one of the important factors that shapes physical activity patterns among children. In the United States, young children cannot travel for long distances by themselves because they cannot drive, there are no safe and practical transit options for children, and the safety risk from travel by nonmotorized means is high. In a world built around the automobile, children are at a distinct disadvantage. Children are either completely reliant on parents for transportation to many destinations or they are limited to a highly restricted spatial realm consisting of a small number of destinations that are readily and safely accessible by nonmotorized means. Children do not walk or ride their bicycles nearly as much as they used to—children's travel by these modes declined by 40 percent from 1977 to 1995. Walking or bicycling to school, a phenomenon that used to be a ritual for children, is now a rare occurrence. As shown in figure 5-1, the percentage of American children who walked to school in 1995 was estimated to be only around 10 percent, whereas thirty years ago the percentage was closer to half of all children (National Safe Kids Campaign 2002). Even for school trips of less than one mile, only 31 percent were made on foot and fewer than 2 percent were by bicycle (FHWA 1997). Other survey data have confirmed these

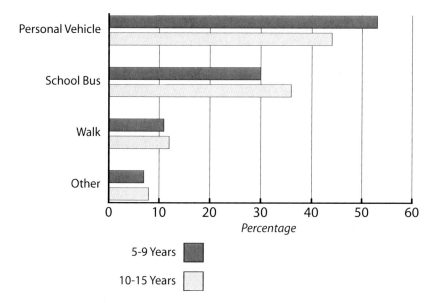

FIGURE 5-1. Percent of children's home-to-school trips by mode, United States, 1995.
Source: Federal Highway Administration 1997.

generally low rates of walking and bicycling to school. A national study conducted by the CDC reported that in 1999 about 11 percent of all trips to school were on foot with another 3 percent reported as being by bicycle (CDC 2002a). These statistics are repeated at the state level as well; a study in Georgia reported that only *4 percent* of children in the state walked to school on the majority of schooldays in 2000 (CDC 2002b).

Children may be less mobile now because of heightened environmental barriers to their independent travel. There appear to be two primary barriers facing children in the contemporary environment: distance between destinations and traffic safety. The 1999 CDC national survey of households (cited in the above paragraph) also asked adults whether their children faced obstacles getting to school on foot or by bicycle. The results, shown in figure 5-2, indicate that distance to school was the biggest obstacle (55 percent of all respondents indicated this as a barrier) followed by traffic dangers (40 percent). Only 16 percent of all respondents indicated that there were no barriers (CDC 2002a).[2]

The CDC results regarding parents' concerns is a finding consistent with other studies of parental fears for their children's travel safety (Davis 1998; Daisa, Jones, and Wachtel 1996). Parents seem to apply these fears especially

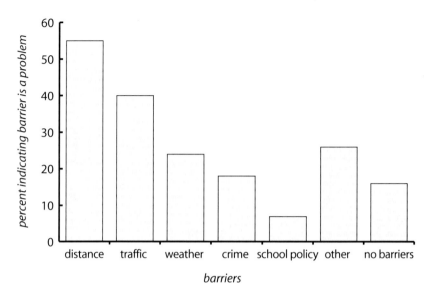

FIGURE 5-2. Parents' perceptions of barriers to their children's travel to school on foot or by bicycle, United States, 1999. Source: HealthStyles Survey, as reported in CDC 2002a.

to younger children. In the 1999 CDC survey, many more adults indicated that traffic danger was a barrier for younger children (aged 5–11 years) than to older ones (aged 12–18 years). These concerns are not misplaced: the number of accidents involving children is a significant percentage of all pedestrian-automobile accidents in many countries, the United States included (OECD 1998). One study of childhood injury-related deaths, for example, revealed that of some 22,000 such deaths in the United States between 1980 and 1985, 37 percent involved motor vehicles. Of these, one-half of the children were fatally injured while walking or bicycling (Waller, Barker, and Szocka 1989). The design of the built environment is a heavy contributor to a large number of accidents involving child pedestrians. Street designs that allow for heavy traffic volumes and high vehicle speeds, for example, tend to produce more accidents involving child pedestrians (Roberts et al. 1995).

Younger children are more vulnerable to traffic hazards because they possess unique attributes that make their travel in the built environment more difficult and dangerous than that of adults. Children process environmental cues differently than adults and, as a result, have difficulty making sound decisions with respect to negotiating that environment. For example, their attention spans tend to be shorter and they tend to have more difficulty in grasping complex traffic rules and situations (Appleyard 1981). Besides these cognitive issues, children also possess different physical characteristics than adults. They are smaller, which prevents them from seeing over tall objects such as parked cars or shrubbery. This means that it is harder for the child to see traffic conditions on a street that they are attempting to cross or to negotiate and harder for the driver to spot the child, particularly when the view of the child is partially or completely obstructed by an object. Both of these problems are compounded by the fact that children simply have less experience in dealing with traffic than adults. All of the subtle understandings of driver behavior that an adult has built up through years of experience are absent in the younger child's mind.

An interesting hypothesis is that parents, knowing that their children are particularly vulnerable to traffic hazards, make decisions that dramatically affect the amount and types of physical activity that they allow their children to get. To protect them from being injured or killed in traffic, parents place restrictions on their children's travel, which in turn decreases the amount of physical activity that they get through the course of their day. In this formulation, parents have the power to grant or withhold "licenses" that permit their children to travel by themselves in the built environment. A more lenient license is given when a parent believes that the child will be safe when traveling alone or with peers; a more restrictive license is imposed when the parent believes that the environment is too unsafe for travel that is unaccompanied by an adult.

This thesis has received a good deal of attention in Europe. In 1990, three British researchers published a major study on the subject of parental constraints on children's travel (Hillman, Adams, and Whitelegg 1990). They explored the travel patterns and levels of personal autonomy of English and German children aged 7–11 and 11–15 years. The authors began by focusing on a statistic that would seem to indicate that the world is reasonably safe for nonmotorized travel by children: the fatality rates in Britain from accidents between motor vehicles and child pedestrians dropped substantially between the late 1970s and late 1980s. Yet these statistics, the authors believed, were misleading: they did not account for the frequency with which children were exposed to traffic danger. If, they speculated, children were traveling less frequently on their own on foot or by bicycle, thereby decreasing their exposure to traffic, fatality statistics could not be interpreted as showing that the built environment was becoming increasingly safe for children. Rather, these statistics would simply reflect a reduction in the amount of nonmotorized travel by children.

Using data from published sources as well as from their own surveys of schoolchildren, the authors of this study found that British children were allowed to travel on their own consistently less than German children. The authors speculated that the differences in travel rates between these countries could be explained by a number of social and cultural factors. However, they also placed great emphasis upon differences in the built environment between German and British cities. German cities had higher population densities and better public transportation systems, conditions that both shortened distances between destinations for children and also gave children a safe and practical means—transit—to reach destinations that were too far away to reach on foot or by bicycle. Moreover, the density of facilities was far greater in the German cities that were studied than in the British ones; playgrounds, parks, and schools were closer to more children and, therefore, much more accessible to German children on foot or by bicycle.[3] For British children, moreover, the study found that fewer children were allowed to travel by themselves in 1990 than in 1971, when a similar study was conducted (table 5-2). The withdrawal of parental permission to walk or bike to school or other destinations in Britain was accompanied by a shift from walking and public transportation to the automobile. More than 40 percent of the British parents who were interviewed as part of the study listed traffic danger as the reason given for restricting the younger children (ages 7–11) from coming home alone after school. By way of contrast, only about 20 percent said their children were unreliable or they feared molestation by strangers and only about 15 percent said the distance home from school was too great. This finding should be contrasted with the results shown in figure 5-2 from the 1999 CDC study in the United States, where parents identified distance the most frequently and traffic danger the second-most frequently.

CHILDREN AND RECREATIONAL PHYSICAL ACTIVITY

Utilitarian travel is not the only way that the built environment is relevant to children's activity patterns. It also influences children's physical activity patterns in terms of recreational physical activity. Because children have a

TABLE 5-2
Loss of childhood mobility in Britain

	1971	1990
7–11 year olds allowed to travel to and from school on their own	86%	29%
Children allowed to cross the road on their own (7–11 years)	72%	51%
Children allowed to take public transportation on their own	48%	15%

SOURCE: Hillman, Adams, Whitelegg: *One False Move . . . A Study of Children's Independent Mobility* (1990), Tables 1, 4, Appendix 3. Reproduced with permission of the Policy Studies Institute, London.

large amount of free time, and because peer groups are very important to childhood development, children get much of their physical activity from playing with other children in social settings outdoors. Sound physical, emotional, and social development may depend on this kind of healthy interaction with other children in play settings. The built environment therefore provides a critical forum for this type of physical activity.

Many have long viewed playgrounds as providing the necessary spaces for children's play, leading to a widespread belief that they should be an integral component of neighborhood design. This basic idea formed a critical part of the design of Clarence Perry's Neighborhood Unit in the 1920s, for example, and also became a central feature of Clarence Stein's designs of the late 1930s. However, streets have always been attractive areas for children's play as well, the integration of playgrounds into neighborhoods notwithstanding. Despite the obvious attractiveness of playgrounds for facilitating play, some argue that they will never be able to fully meet children's needs with respect to play in the built environment. This argument is based on the observation that children's play is often an unstructured activity that occurs in spontaneous ways and places. Robin Moore, a landscape architect who specializes in designing environments for children, has argued that while children do make substantial use of playgrounds for play, streets often serve as even more attractive playgrounds, of sorts, for children (Moore 1987). Streets are valued by children in large part because they are so proximate to children's homes: they are close enough so that travel time to and from the play space is limited, a factor that is crucial when considering that children's lives are guided by time constraints that are established by their parents. Streets are available as play areas during those often brief periods when children are not obliged to be anywhere or doing anything, such as between the end of the school day and dinner and between dinner and sundown. Therefore, according to Moore, streets are important social areas for children, places that are easily accessible for meetings. They are amongst the few environments children have that are relatively free of play rules—parents often constrain noise and types of play in enclosed backyards. Finally, streets are often more interesting spaces than playgrounds. The areas on and along streets offer a host of features that, to a child, offer up an endless variety of opportunities for creative play and imagination. These features include curbs, gutters, sidewalks, trees, parked cars, fences, mailboxes, walls, and interesting passersby.

For decades, a part of the suburban ideal has been that the suburb offers the kind of safe, low-traffic streets that children need in order to be safe. The cul-de-sac is now the dominant type of street in residential subdivisions in part because parents view these streets as providing safe havens for their children. The reason for its current popularity is the same as that expressed by Clarence Stein when he laid out his Radburn street network: the street that is detached from through-traffic is safe for children because it diverts traffic away from local streets and slows the speed of cars entering the street. Whether or not such claims are accurate, there is a perverse consequence of developing residential subdivisions in this way. For children, practical travel becomes much more difficult. When many streets are dead-ends, getting from home to school or friends' houses often requires a much longer trip because there is no direct way to go from point A to point B (this concept is discussed more fully in chapter 7). This has the effect of reducing children's travel on foot or by bicycle because distances between destinations such as home and school increase, often dramatically. In addition, the cul-de-sac arrangement forces traffic onto high-speed arterials along the edges of neighborhoods, making pedestrian or bicyclist travel along and across such streets highly dangerous, especially for children.

Unfortunately, contemporary development patterns limit children's spatial horizons. Low population densities and dangerous crossings of the arterials that run between neighborhoods make it difficult for children to reach a large number of other children's houses by themselves. Schools, too, are so far away that children often have no way of getting there without being driven by their parents or taking a bus. When purchasing a house in a leafy subdivision, parents are attempting to shelter and protect their children and to enhance their children's play by giving them a safe environment. The consequence, however, may be to dampen their overall levels of physical activity by making journeys on foot or by bicycle nearly impossible.

The Elderly

The elderly are one of the fastest growing demographic groups in the United States and, indeed, within all of the world's wealthiest countries. As noted, people aged sixty-five and older comprise about 12 percent of the American population, a figure that will grow as the Baby Boomers reach retirement age. There has been much discussion of the profound effect that this demographic transition will have on American political, social, and economic life. It remains to be seen whether the elderly will also play a major role in reshaping the built environment to suit their needs as diminished capabilities begin to reduce their ability to move about safely on their own. The aging process generates a number of problems that hinder the full range of physical capabilities most people enjoy during their early adulthood and that contribute to their ability and desire to engage in certain activities in the built environment. The list of aging-related problems includes chronic pain from arthritis and rheumatism, reduced muscle and bone mass, declining sensory perception (deterioration of vision and hearing), and slower reflexes. Some elderly people face eroded mental capabilities, the result of dementia (e.g., Alzheimer's disease) or other diseases. An even greater percentage may experience more generalized signs of psychological difficulties, such as a lower stress threshold and a reduced desire to interact with the larger environment in which they live (Fitzpatrick and LaGory 2000).

Regular physical activity is believed to play an important role in countering many of these physical and mental health problems. Physical activity maintains good health in the elderly or at least delays the onset of many negative health conditions. Physical activity, for example, delays disabilities from osteoporosis and other conditions. If engaged in over the course of one's adult years, physical activity may also delay the onset of chronic disease. Finally, regular physical activity in the form of walking or other moderate activities may alleviate depression in the elderly and improve their quality of life. Walking within one's community may generate psychological benefits due to an increase in social interaction.

As was mentioned in chapter 3, national health data show that physical activity levels decline with age, which in the American context is quite dramatic (table 5-3). To some degree, of course, this is as expected. As people age, they face a lengthening list of health problems that hinder their ability to get enough physical activity. Additionally, for many middle-aged adults, aging means more work and family responsibilities and less time for leisure-time physical activity. Finally, the aging process seems to produce physiological changes that make people less energetic as the years and decades pass. When combined, these factors must account for much of the abysmally low rates of physical activity for people in the last third or quarter of their lives. Yet, these factors cannot tell the entire story of declining physical activity for the elderly; work and family responsibilities generally lessen, to give one example, after a person retires and once children have left home. Moreover, data from other countries suggest that elderly people do not have to be as inactive as data from the United States suggest that they are. These and other considerations indicate, therefore, that the environments in which the elderly live and run their lives must also serve to constrain activity patterns.

The elderly face multiple difficulties with respect to physical activity in the built environment. As with children, the elderly generally find that their ability to engage in recreational and utilitarian forms of physical activity in the built environment is more constrained than younger adults. While the reasons vary depending on each individual's health status, all have to do with the effects of age on the elderly person's ability to safely and quickly negotiate the built environment. The elderly frequently have some erosion of one or more physical capabilities, such as the loss of eyesight and hearing or the deterioration of one's sense of balance, resulting in changed perceptions of, and behavior in, the built environment. The consequence is that the elderly tend to skew their travel patterns around safety considerations to an extent that is greater than younger adults. The elderly rely upon the car for a large percentage of all trips, just like younger adults—nationwide data show that more than 90 percent of all trips made by this group are by car (FHWA 1997). Many elderly people view travel by car as being a positive, for the car is believed to provide levels of security, comfort, and convenience that other forms of transportation in the United States are not perceived to provide. Alternatives to the

TABLE 5-3
Physical activity by age group, United States, 2000

	18–24 years,	25–44 years	45–64 years	65–74 years	75 and over
Active*	40%	35%	30%	27%	16%
Sedentary**	31%	34%	41%	46%	59%

*Defined as engaging in sufficient moderate (min. 5 times/week for 30 minutes a day) and/or vigorous (min. 3 times/week for 20 minutes a day) physical activity to meet public health guidelines.
**Defined as no leisure-time physical activity.
SOURCE: "Data 2010: The Healthy People 2010 Database," Focus Area 22. Available online at http://198.246.96.90/HP2010/INDEX.HTM.

automobile tend to be viewed with some suspicion by the elderly, particularly by those who live in suburban areas. Transit is seen as being a potentially dangerous form of travel, as many elderly report being harassed by strangers, or at least the fear of being harassed by strangers, while taking transit. Some studies report that the elderly are victims of crime while taking transit more frequently than other adults, and the elderly themselves report a higher fear of crime with respect to transit (Coughlin 2001; Wachs 1988). Transportation studies also repeatedly show that the elderly take fewer trips overall, by car as well as other modes, compared with younger adults. While some of this is due to the obvious fact that most elderly people are retired and thus no longer commute to work, the consensus is that the elderly make fewer trips because they fear the problems and dangers involved in travel, an observation that is not constrained to the United States (OECD 1998).

These fears overlap with concerns that the elderly have about walking, having to do with the ways that the built environment creates dangers for the elderly pedestrian. In large sections of American cities, walking is impractical for the elderly, just as it is for other adults and children, given long distances between destinations. In cases where distances are not too great, however, safety considerations seem to be especially important in influencing the willingness of the elderly to walk to a destination. High-speed traffic, incomplete sidewalk networks, and other attributes of the built environment contribute to the perception amongst the elderly that it is unsafe for the pedestrian. In many instances electronic crosswalk signals at street intersections are timed for younger people, who walk at speeds higher than many elderly are capable of going (Coughlin and Lacombe 1997).[4]

The elderly span all economic, social, ethnic, and racial lines. The term "elderly" also encompasses several age strata, from the relatively youthful

[89]

(perhaps sixty-five to seventy-four years) to older (perhaps seventy-five to eighty-five years) and very old ages. The elderly are spatially well distributed, both in terms of distribution across the United States and within cities and regions. Perhaps three quarters of the elderly population live in low-density suburban or nonmetropolitan areas (Coughlin and Lacombe 1997). While there is considerable demographic heterogeneity within the elderly suburban population, in general they tend to be wealthier than the elderly population living in central cities. For the suburban elderly, recreational physical activity may be fairly easy to come by, as residential subdivisions generally have quiet local streets that are relatively safe for strolling. The problem for this group involves physical activity for utilitarian purposes as well as for recreational purposes at facilities outside of their own neighborhoods—getting to a park or shopping district may be very difficult due to the ways that the built environment creates barriers for them. (The suburban elderly do, however, often walk in environments that are highly controlled and safe environments, such as indoor malls). Moreover, the suburban elderly are as dependent upon the automobile for meeting practical transportation needs as other adults in the suburbs, perhaps more so because they have even fewer transportation alternatives available to them, due to physical limitations that can impede non-motorized travel and even the use of transit. As many observers point out, for the suburban elderly, travel by car becomes increasingly problematic as one advances in age. Inevitably, all, or nearly all, members of this group face the problem of being unable to drive at some point during their retirement years.

In contrast, a higher percentage of the elderly who live in more urbanized areas do not own or operate automobiles, in many instances due to lower incomes. This group must face the question of travel without access to their own automobile at an earlier age. Fortunately, alternative forms of transportation in central cities tend to be more readily available, and distances between destinations are shorter. As a result, the urban elderly should have more opportunity for utilitarian physical activity. (Interestingly, data from a study conducted in the Atlanta region showed that elderly residents located in communities with higher densities may be more active and, thus, healthier as a result—they were on average five pounds leaner than those who lived in lower density neighborhoods.)[5] Nonetheless, the urban elderly simultaneously may face numerous problems with respect to utilitarian travel, facing issues relating to personal security and convenience when using transit, get-

ting to and from transit stops, and the safety of walking in the built environment in general (Wachs 1988).

ELDERLY PHYSICAL ACTIVITY PATTERNS—INTERNATIONAL EVIDENCE

Data from other countries provide support for the argument that the built
environment can have a positive influence on physical activity patterns
amongst the elderly, as opposed to the negative role it seems to play in the
United States. Walking constitutes a significant mode of transportation in
most wealthy countries, the United States excepted, and is perhaps even more
popular amongst the elderly than among younger adults in other countries.
A 1995 national travel survey in Great Britain, for example, found that walking accounted for 36 percent of all journeys by elderly men and 40 percent by
elderly women, compared to 19 percent of younger men's journeys and 27
percent of younger female's journeys. In New Zealand, a 1991 survey found
that 33 percent of journeys made by people aged seventy and over were made
on foot, compared to 16 percent for adults between twenty-five and fifty-nine
(OECD 1998). Perhaps the most astonishing comparative data is provided in
table 5-4, which compares the travel patterns of the elderly in the Netherlands, Germany, and the United States. Fully a quarter of all trips by the
Dutch elderly are by bicycle, an astonishing figure, especially when compared
with the figure for the United States (0.2 percent). The figure for bicycling is
lower for Germany but still much higher than in the U.S. Moreover, the figures for walking are extremely high in both European countries (19–24
percent in the Netherlands and 39–48 percent in Germany) compared to
the United States (6 percent). Given that the Netherlands and Germany are
wealthy countries (e.g., many people can afford to own and operate a car), the
only plausible explanation for such large disparities across these countries is
the influence of cultural attitudes and values as well as the effect that the built
environment has on the willingness of people to engage in utilitarian physical activity. Many Dutch and German cities have gone to great lengths over
the past few decades to enhance and expand bicycling and pedestrian facilities as well as to change traffic laws for the protection of nonmotorists (these
measures are discussed in chapters 7 and 9). When coupled with existing land
use patterns and urban design characteristics of Dutch and German cities,
these investments seem to have made travel by nonmotorized means, and
bicycling in particular, an attractive option for many elderly people. This state

of affairs should be contrasted with the United States, where a discussion of utilitarian bicycling and walking by the elderly is almost completely off the public's agenda.

The Poor

The linkage between low-income status (and related indicators of low income including lower educational attainment and minority status) and negative health outcomes is well established. Being poor is associated with a higher risk of mortality, contracting a chronic disease, becoming overweight or obese, or suffering from some other health problem (CDC 1999a; Mokdad et al. 1999; Fiscella and Franks 1997). Moreover, research shows that poor health results from both low income and also the environment in which one lives. Poor people fare better in middle-class neighborhoods than do their counterparts in neighborhoods where the majority of people are poor. In other words, a high concentration of poverty appears to have an independent influence on health, even after taking into account the income status of each indi-

TABLE 5-4

*Modal split (% of all trips taken by mode) for
the elderly in the Netherlands, Germany, and
the United States*

	Age group	
	65–74	75+
Netherlands		
Automobile	51	43
Transit	4	7
Bicycle	25	24
Walking	19	24
Germany		
Automobile	35	21
Transit	15	24
Bicycle	11	7
Walking	39	48
United States*		
Automobile	91	
Transit	2	
Bicycle	0.2	
Walking	6	

*Figures available only from age 65 and older.
SOURCE: John Pucher and Lewis Dijkstra, "Making Walking and Cycling Safer: Lessons from Europe," *Transportation Quarterly*, 2000, Vol 54, No. 3, pp. 25–50. Reprinted with permission of *Transportation Quarterly*, Eno Transportation Foundation, Washington, DC.

TABLE 5-5.
Physical inactivity by income level, United States, 1992

Annual household income	Percent sedentary
<$10,000	41.5
$10,000–$20,000	34.6
$20,000–$35,000	26.9
$35,000–$50,000	23.0
>$50,000	17.7

*Data from the 1992 Behavioral Risk Factor Surveillance System (BRFSS).
SOURCE: U.S. Department of Health and Human Services 1996, Table 5-2.

vidual living there (Balfour and Kaplan 2002; Waitzman and Smith 1998; Ellaway, Anderson, and Macintyre 1997). This logic extends to physical activity as well: living in a poorer area seems to have a dampening effect on physical activity, independent of the poverty status of individual residents (Yen and Kaplan 1998).

Indeed, as shown in table 5-5, lower incomes and physical inactivity tend to go hand-in-hand. People who are poor may face a more formidable combination of personal and environmental barriers to physical activity than those faced by people with higher incomes. They may face greater personal barriers, for instance, because they may have less leisure time available to them, have little in the way of discretionary income that allows them to engage in some types of physical activity, or may not have adequate information about the amounts and types of physical activity that are necessary to maintain good health. Environmental barriers to recreational physical activity are also problematic for low-income individuals, as poorer neighborhoods are likely to contain fewer amenities such as sports fields. However, how the environment influences and shapes utilitarian physical activity for members of this group is a bit more complicated.

Because auto ownership rates are lower for low-income households than for higher-income ones, the poor have a much greater difficulty in reaching all destinations within a region, including the full range of employment, commercial, retail, entertainment, and even personal destinations. Nationwide, poorer households make 20 percent fewer trips than wealthier households, and they travel only half as far in terms of vehicle miles traveled (Murakami and Young 1997). This problem is acute for many minority groups as well, in particular low-income minority groups, who travel fewer miles per day on average, make fewer automobile trips and more transit and walk trips

TABLE 5-6.
Travel patterns by racial/ethnic status, United States

	African American	Hispanic	Caucasian
Person miles of travel	31	4	41
Vehicle trips (as driver)	722	820	1,006
Transit trips	95	48	15
Walk trips	131	126	72

SOURCES: U.S. Department of Transportation 1999, figure 3; Federal Highway Administration 1997, figures 27 and 28.

(table 5-6). These statistics, of course, simply reflect the fact that members of lower-income (and lower-income minority) groups who live in metropolitan areas tend to live in higher density areas that are nearer to transit service, resulting in the need to travel fewer miles to reach *some* destinations. These statistics also, however, underscore a basic accessibility problem—poorer residents of cities travel less in part because they cannot access *all* destinations within a region.

Therefore, the poor must rely upon transit and nonmotorized travel for a greater share of trips than the rest of the population. While this is good from the standpoint of physical activity, there are significant problems with respect to how easy and safe it is for poor people to negotiate the built environment while walking, bicycling, or using transit. First, these alternative modes do not make up the accessibility deficit for the poor. Transit rarely, if ever, services an entire region; transit provision is notoriously bad in most suburban growth areas, where many jobs and services are clustered. The prospects for walking and bicycling are often not much better. Most recent suburban development simply makes distances too great to make walking and bicycling practical forms of travel. Second, and more importantly from a public health perspective, the use of alternative modes by the poor entails a high risk of physical danger. Accident statistics between motorists and pedestrians generally show that the poor suffer a disproportionate number of injuries and fatalities while walking than do members of wealthier groups. As many streets tend to be engineered with the motorist in mind, those who rely upon nonmotorized modes of travel often have no choice but to follow very dangerous routes in order to get to school, shopping, or work. Children from disadvantaged backgrounds, for example, are at a much higher risk for injury than are children from more privileged backgrounds. While it is not clear whether this is due to greater traffic volumes near where poorer children live, the absence of parks and playgrounds near these children's homes, or the result of more exposure to traffic (lower income children may have to walk more due to the fewer number of automobiles in lower income households), the fact is that lower-income children, and especially children of lower-income minorities, are injured and killed more often while walking and bicycling than are children from more affluent families (Durkin et al. 1999; Forkenbrock and Schweitzer 1997; Durkin et al. 1994; Pless et al. 1987).

THE POOR AND PHYSICAL ACTIVITY: ATLANTA

These problems are exemplified by the situation that confronts the poor in one of the nation's largest metropolitan regions, Atlanta. During the 1980s and 1990s, the Atlanta region experienced some of the fastest growth rates in the United States, adding some 1.2 million people during the 1990s alone. The bulk of this growth was in the northern half of the region, with the most intense development occurring at the urban periphery and within suburban activity centers. Unfortunately, as is the case in many American cities, a large fraction of the region's poor are concentrated in neighborhoods that did not share in the region's growth, in areas surrounding the downtown and extending southward from downtown. The nature of Atlanta's growth has therefore created a gap between where the bulk of the region's jobs are located and where most of the region's poor reside (Bullard, Johnson, and Torres 2000). To make things worse, Atlanta's growth during the 1980s and 1990s dramatically reduced what was an already low population density level for the entire region. According to land use statistics issued by the Brookings Institution, in 1982 the region had a population density of 3.2 persons per urbanized acre. By 1997, the region's 3.6 million people required 1.3 million acres of urbanized land, resulting in an average density of 2.8 people per urbanized acre. As a result, the region ranks third in the United States in terms of lowest population density, behind only Nashville and Charlotte (Fulton et al. 2001).

Atlanta's growth therefore produced conditions that made it much more difficult for the poor to access jobs and services by way of transit or nonmotorized means, because such densities meant that only a small number of destinations were within walking distance from a typical transit stop. Walking for utilitarian purposes without relying on transit is made even more difficult in Atlanta by the fact that proposition, as there are few areas of concentrated employment and services that are near poor neighborhoods. Of these, most are located in the center of the region. Compounding this problem in

Atlanta is the fact that the region's transit system, MARTA, provides rail service for only two core counties, which together account for only a fraction of the region's population.[6] The rail system services a limited area even within these counties, as it is a simple pattern consisting of only two major routes that cross at a single point—this layout reflects MARTA's origins as a system designed to speed commuters into downtown from outlying suburbs. Many of the region's outlying counties either have no bus service at all or have just begun implementation of bus systems. Yet despite the limited reach of the region's transit systems, Atlanta's poor households must rely upon them to provide access to many jobs and services. About three quarters of MARTA's riders are members of a racial and ethnic minority, and four out of five live in the region's core counties. A major barrier to economic opportunity for these groups is therefore considered to be the yawning spatial divide between many of the region's employment centers and its housing for the region's poor (Bullard, Johnson, and Torres 2000).

An equally important issue, pedestrian safety, accompanies these problems for Atlanta's poor. A study of pedestrian fatality rates in four metropolitan Atlanta counties by the CDC found that rates for African Americans and Hispanics were two and six times greater, respectively, than rates for whites (CDC 1999c). While the CDC observed, quite correctly, that members of these groups also walk more frequently than whites, the finding nonetheless supports the proposition that the Atlanta transportation system is particularly unsafe for minorities and, especially, for lower-income minorities who are unable to afford a private vehicle. These observations are bolstered by anecdotal information about areas of the Atlanta region that are particularly dangerous for low-income pedestrians. Buford Highway, for example, is a major thoroughfare that stretches northeast from the region's core. Dominated by high-speed and high-volume traffic, like most major thoroughfares in Atlanta and around the country, Buford Highway is simply not designed for pedestrian travel and few people would willingly choose to walk along it or to cross over it. There are few sidewalks, well-marked crosswalks, pedestrian refuges, street trees, or any other features that make pedestrian travel safe and enjoyable. Yet people walk along Buford Highway, despite its lack of pedestrian amenities, generating some of the highest pedestrian accident rates in the region (photo 5-1). The reason why so many people walk along and try to cross over the highway is that the residential areas surrounding it

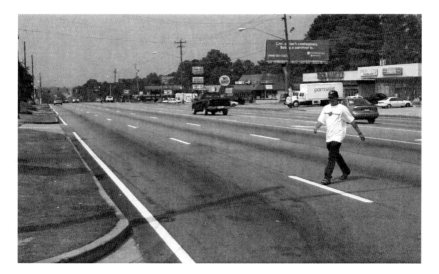

PHOTO 5-1. Buford Highway is one of the most dangerous streets for walking in the Atlanta region. Pedestrians, many of whom are low-income Hispanics, must negotiate seven lanes of high-speed traffic, frequently without a crosswalk or other facilities that might make such crossings safer.

are home to a large percentage of the region's low-income Hispanic population, who consequently make up the bulk of the pedestrian injuries and fatalities along the highway. Unfortunately, the residents of the area have no choice but to travel along Buford Highway, and to cross over it at unsafe mid-block crossings, in order to reach necessary destinations.

Conclusion

This chapter has shown that the built environment's influence on physical activity should not be discussed without reference to people who suffer from physical and economic disadvantages. Unfortunately for the poor, children, and the elderly, most environments are not constructed with their limitations uppermost in mind. Many environments that seem to middle-aged, healthy, and affluent people as fully usable may not be so for people who face a multitude of problems. The worst-off groups in society suffer the most in environments built around the needs of motorists. The combined effect of being poor and either very young or very old, for example, is profound; these individuals suffer the most from the barriers created by environments built without their needs in mind. The significance of differentiating between different groups has to do with the insights that can be gained with respect to the design of the built environment for encouraging physical activity. The design and arrangement of nearly everything in the built environment—buildings, parking lots, transit facilities, sidewalks, crosswalks—has equity implications. When the built environment is designed to meet the needs of the typical or average person, which in American parlance has come to be equated with the motorist, other groups usually suffer. Environments that encourage utilitarian physical activity are also those environments that will present the fewest barriers to the members of disadvantaged groups.

CHAPTER SIX

Understanding the Built Environment

In this chapter and the three following chapters, we attempt to make sense of the built environment's influence on physical activity by breaking the built environment down into three basic components—transportation systems, land use patterns, and urban design characteristics. The purpose of this chapter is to sketch an outline of why each component is important and also to discuss some of the major obstacles that stand in the way of understanding how each component influences physical activity. The following three chapters are devoted to detailing the individual components, which shape the built environment in fundamental ways through: locating key origins and destinations within space (housing, offices, shopping, recreational destinations), determining the ease and type of access between these origins and destinations, establishing the safety of different types of spaces (streets, sidewalks, parks, plazas) for different users, and influencing the basic desirability of being in those spaces in the first place. When appropriate, we discuss how the components have differential effects with respect to individual types of physical activity. Our remarks tend to be confined to differences between walking and bicycling, as these are two of the most common types of physical activity in the built environment and also provide the means for utilitarian travel. While we break down and analyze each element for its individual contribution to physical activity, it must be emphasized that these components do not exist in isolation one from another. The world that we live in can seem chaotic but in many respects its elements are related in a coherent way—as will be made clear, these components logically overlap with one another.

Transportation systems result from aggregate public and, much more rarely, private investment in transportation infrastructure within a region. Transportation systems can be defined in part as the network of physical infrastructure within a region, such as its street network, its transit systems, and separated systems for nonmotorized users such as jogging and biking paths. However, it can also be defined in mode-specific terms, for example the total infrastructure dedicated to bicycles, which would include both on- and off-street facilities. Transportation systems determine how well destinations are connected to each other. They do this in two ways. First, a transportation network can provide many or few links between places, which will help to determine both how far one has to travel to reach a destination as well as determining how many route options one has to choose from. A "highly connected" street network is one that has many possible routes between destinations, which, almost by definition, means that the trip between any two destinations is reasonably direct. One way to think about this is the difference between the straight-line distance between two destinations (the "crow fly" distance) and the distance over the street network (the "network" distance). A high connectivity network minimizes this difference—if one were to divide the crow fly distance by the network distance (figure 6-1), high connectivity networks would have a ratio closer to one than low connectivity systems. Second, transportation systems can be continuous or fragmented. Continuous systems are those where each part of the system is connected to every other part, forming a seamless network—road systems are the perfect example. Fragmented systems are those where the parts of the system are disconnected from one another, meaning that one cannot travel over the course of the entire network without getting off at some point and traversing some other transportation system. Pedestrian networks, for instance, are almost always fragmented, meaning that the sidewalk system will abruptly end at one place and then begin again one, two, or even many blocks later.

The second component of the built environment consists of land use patterns. These patterns consist of the spatial arrangement of structures on the landscape. How and where residential, commercial, and industrial structures are arrayed define the basic land use patterns within a particular area, which are relevant for travel because they shape the degree of proximity between places across urban space. In other words, they determine how close destinations are to one another, independent of how well or poorly the street network connects the destinations. There are, of course, many ways in which

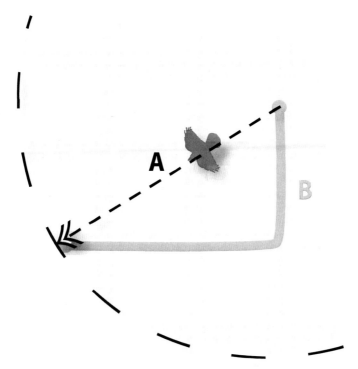

FIGURE 6-1. "Crow-fly" versus "network" distances. The crow-fly distance in this example is illustrated by line A, which is the straight-line distance between two points. The network distance is illustrated by line B, which is the shortest distance that one can travel *along the street network* between the two points.

urbanized land could be categorized, but for our purposes we divide land into two major categories, by density and mixture of uses. Density gauges how compact the built environment is, and is measured in a number of different ways, both in terms of people as well as structures. It is generally accepted that higher densities of people are associated with higher structural densities (the number of buildings distributed over a given spatial area, basically a measure of the intensity of building in a part of a city). As a result, higher density levels are believed to reduce trip lengths, thereby increasing travel options (walking, bicycling, and transit) as well as obviating the need to own a vehicle (Frank and Pivo 1995). There are some difficulties with this concept. For example, scholars disagree regarding how to define density with precision and over which geographic scale to measure the concept. Density also might serve to conceal other urban form or demographic factors that are at work and that, perhaps, are more important in explaining why people behave the way they do. Regardless of these critiques, few dismiss the idea that, at some level, density is an indispensable requirement for shortening distances between activities while simultaneously making transit easier to use and more feasible for the transit provider.

Land use mix, the second land use variable of interest, refers to the degree to which different types of uses (residential, commercial, retail) are located within close proximity to one another. Most suburban development is characterized by single uses (e.g., housing is separated from commercial development, which in turn is separated from retail development). Single uses are believed to increase trip lengths and auto ownership and decrease transit usage for the journey to work (Cervero 1988). As with density, mixing uses increases proximity (shortens trip distances), thereby increasing the likelihood that alternative forms of transportation, in particular walking, bicycling, and transit, are viable. Mixed use can be measured both in terms of vertical and horizontal mix. Vertical mix occurs when different land uses are stacked one upon another, such as housing located over commercial or retail establishments. Horizontal mix is when different land uses are located within close proximity to each other—these uses are mixed together, as the term implies.

Together, transportation systems and land use patterns account for much of the variability within and between cities around the world, at least at the very coarse spatial levels at which these concepts tend to be measured (at finer or smaller spatial levels, these concepts do less well in differentiating between places). These components work together to define the basic spatial parameters of a place within the built environment. As shown in table 6-1, a place can exhibit one of four basic patterns that result from this interaction. It can have either high or low connectivity, and either high or low proximity. Development that is high in connectivity and high in proximity (the upper left-hand cell) used to be quite common in the United States—many older neighborhoods, in particular those built in the early twentieth century along trolley lines, possess such a combination—and is still fairly common in many cities elsewhere in the world. At the other extreme (the lower right-hand cell) is development that is low in connectivity and low in proximity. This type of development characterizes many, if not most, areas of cities in the United States that have been built over the past half-century. However, it is impor-

TABLE 6-1
Built environment matrix, by connectivity and proximity

	High connectivity	Low connectivity
High proximity	Traditional neighborhoods	Adjacent uses in suburbs
Low proximity	High-income residential enclaves in urban centers	Contemporary suburban development

tant to note that low connectivity and high proximity development (the upper right-hand box in table 6-1) is also common and exists in many suburban areas of the nation. In this land use pattern, residential development is located in close proximity to retail and commercial development, but there is little opportunity for direct travel between these uses. In such cases, roadways seldom directly connect different adjacent uses (and, indeed, even adjacent developments that fall into the same land use category, such as adjoining residential subdivisions). To make matters worse, walls and other obstacles are frequently inserted between adjoining uses to prevent people from walking between the two. Many commercial offices and retail shopping centers, for example, are located adjacent to large-scale and high-density apartment complexes, yet again the internal circulation systems, and connections to adjacent developments, make it impossible to move directly from one development to another. The final type of development, consisting of high connectivity and low-density development (the lower left-hand cell of table 6-1) is found to a more limited extent in older, more established and affluent residential enclaves within urban centers. Here, residential subdivisions near the urban core were built for the wealthy during an early wave of suburban development. They are low in density, often consisting of large houses on large lots, yet they are relatively high in connectivity because their street systems are not as disconnected as newer development.

Finally, urban design characteristics influence how an individual perceives the built environment. In making a decision about whether or not to walk or bicycle, people will factor into their decision not only considerations related to distance and accessibility—how close destinations are to each other as well as how easy it is to reach them by a particular mode—but also a slew of intangibles as well, including safety and attractiveness. The number and width of traffic lanes, the type of pavement used for surfacing, the location and marking of crosswalks, the size and extensiveness of sidewalks, and the type and siting of miscellaneous objects on and around the street—tree plantings, benches, and so forth—all come into play in influencing how a person views the street. Some streets will be more preferable for walking and bicycling than others. Some design treatments will create streets that are better for automobile travel than for nonmotorized travel, and vice versa. An example is traffic calming, which seeks to transform neighborhood roads to reduce the potential for accidents between motorists and nonmotorists, minimize vehicle pollution and noise, and recapture street space for use by nonmotorists. The intent is to redesign the road surface in order to dramatically slow traffic speeds, thereby encouraging alternative forms of travel (Grava 1993). Similarly, the ways that buildings and other elements of the built environment such as parking lots, parks, squares, monuments, and so forth are designed and situated in the built environment are hypothesized as having a powerful influence on behavior.

Understanding the Built Environment: Conceptual and Practical Issues

The built environment is exceedingly complex and, as a result, behavior in that environment is difficult to understand. The topic of physical activity is a case in point. There are a number of conceptual and practical problems with respect to divining the multiple relationships between physical activity and the built environment. Four are discussed in this section.

PHYSICAL ACTIVITY TYPES: DIVERGENT REQUIREMENTS

There are many influences on one's ability and desire to engage in physical activity. These range from personal experience and motivation to larger environmental, social, and even economic reasons. The ways that the built environment influences each type of activity introduce an additional layer of complexity. The ideal environment for a walk to the market will not be exactly the same as that for someone who is interested in going for a jog. Different types of physical activity, in other words, have their own individual requirements with respect to the attributes within the built environment that will encourage the activity. Sometimes, these requirements will be complementary, as in the case where high quality parks containing sports fields are placed in close proximity to housing and connected by pedestrian-friendly streets. Occasionally, different types of physical activity require divergent types of environments, which in turn necessitate different design treatments. Such divergences may be subtle or dramatic, depending on the type of physical activity.

Differences between bicycling and walking, the two types of physical activity that we concentrate much of our attention on in this book, provide a case in point. These types of physical activity are, as we have asserted, the only two types that are utilitarian as well as recreational, meaning that someone can walk or bicycle for practical purposes, such as a trip to the store or work, in addition to outings whose purpose might be exercise or fun. For utilitarian travel, people who want to walk and bicycle have a nearly identical need with respect to the built environment: short distances between destinations are better. Beyond this common requirement, however, things become a little more complicated. Other features of the built environment will influence the pedestrian differently than the bicyclist, and vice versa. Some features that are highly relevant to one type may simply be irrelevant to the other, while other features that make one type of activity more attractive might make the other less so. Pedestrians require good sidewalks and crosswalks, while bicyclists need either specialized bike paths, dedicated on-street bike lanes, or streets without such lanes on which they can ride with relative safety from automobiles. Pedestrian safety and comfort on the sidewalk is enhanced by on-street parking, which acts as a buffer between traffic and the pedestrian; bicyclists don't particularly enjoy riding next to parked cars because of the risk of car doors being opened in front of them. Pedestrians need highly detailed, interesting spaces along their route (store fronts, building facades, so-called "street furniture," etc.); bicyclists do not require such intricate details in order to maintain their attention, due to the speed at which they travel and the need to concentrate on the road and traffic conditions. For recreational bicycling and walking, these divergences may be even more acute. The ideal conditions for recreational bicycling are low-traffic conditions with few stops (stoplights, stop signs), a condition met by only some types of roads and off-road biking/hiking trails (generally speaking, paved systems designed for use by pedestrians, bicyclists, rollerbladers, and other nonmotorized uses). Recreational walking is, on the other hand, best suited to either social environments, wherein people stroll along a pedestrianized street or other type of highly social space, or quiet environments that allow for fast walking for exercise (parks or residential neighborhoods with good sidewalks).

COLLECTIVE EFFECTS

A second problem has to do with how the built environment tends to be organized. Those features of the built environment that create similar types of behavior are most often found bundled together into the same subdivisions, neighborhoods, and districts; for example, high densities, mixed uses, and traditional design characteristics, each one of which is believed to induce more walking, all tend to be found in the same spots on the urban map. That is to say, where it is denser, it also tends to be more mixed in uses and more interconnected. Unfortunately, for this reason, researchers who attempt to understand how each variable impacts physical activity patterns or other behaviors in the built environment face a problem. To understand the individual impact of, say, residential density on walking is difficult because areas with higher levels of density tend to contain other features that also promote walking. For researchers, disentangling the influence of individual features of the built environment on travel behavior has proven to be exceedingly difficult. This is in addition to the more general problem of having to sort out the influences of the built environment from demographic and economic considerations that are also correlated with behavior.

A variety of efforts have been employed to come to grips with this issue. One strategy is to simply focus on one type of urban form component, such as street networks or density, and ignore other considerations. While these studies have the advantage of apparent specificity, they also fail to control for other urban form variables that may be important in determining activity patterns. Another common strategy is for researchers to attempt to assess the effects of combinations of urban form characteristics that are simultaneously present in neighborhoods. In these studies, a quasi-experimental research design is employed, where two groups of neighborhoods are selected based on common sets of design features. Such designs are called "quasi experimental" in recognition of their attempt to isolate the effect of particular factors like residential density or land use mix on a singular phenomenon such as physical activity, without the capacity of random assignment of study participants to control and experimental groups. Social science researchers commonly resort to such study designs due to the complex set of factors that impact human behavior in real-world settings. For example, neighborhoods that have traditional features, such as grid street patterns, high density levels, and so on, are selected and placed in one group; standard suburban neighborhoods are selected and placed in a second group. Travel statistics are gathered and compared for each group, with variations in travel behavior by group allowing the researcher to conclude that different *sets* of urban form characteristics are influencing the travel behavior. On occasion, researchers will attempt to create research designs that control for the individual effects of urban form variables. This is accomplished either through the use of statistical techniques or through quasi-experimental research designs. Finally, case studies of different neighborhoods or transportation improvements are frequently employed. These studies often contain a temporal component, where travel behavior is measured before and after a design change is made to an urban area.

The upshot is that while it is possible to tease out the effects of individual variables of interest on behavior, or at least the influence of clusters of similar variables, research is perennially hampered by the problem of spatial co-variation. There is a good reason as to why this is the case: individual features of the built environment that contribute to making a place more or less friendly to nonmotorized travel complement one another. Architects, landscape architects, and urban designers who are interested in making places that are more pedestrian and bicycling oriented repeatedly underscore the importance of designing places that have multiple reinforcing attributes; anything less results in failure.[1] This is simply inherent to the study of the city, which is one reason why understanding the influence of the built environment on any behavior, travel or otherwise, is always so complicated.

ADDING TRIPS VERSUS REPLACING THEM

An assumption made by those who advocate the shortening of trip distances (by way of improving both proximity and connectivity) is that shorter distances will increase the number of trips taken on foot or by bicycle. This is a wholly reasonable position and has much empirical support. However, some critics of this view hold a contrary position. They argue that the shortening of trip distances will not necessarily result in more trips taken by nonmotorized modes and/or may result in more trips being taken by car.

Randall Crane, a professor at the University of California at Los Angeles, has most forcefully asserted this line of reasoning. Crane argues that those who want to improve connectivity and proximity between destinations (here

Crane directs his critiques specifically at New Urbanists) have failed to construct a theory of travel behavior, accepting on faith the idea that shortening distances between destinations will motivate people to walk and bicycle more while driving less. This reasoning, Crane insists, makes intuitive sense but upon closer analysis may prove to be unfounded. He argues that an individual's decision to make a trip can be represented as a micro-economic problem of benefits weighed against costs. The cost of a trip consists of those things that add hassles to one's day or burdens one's pocketbook: the amount of time it takes to travel, the amount of traffic that might be encountered along the journey, and how much money the trip might require. The choice to drive, take transit, walk, or bicycle is therefore viewed as a function of one's preferences for a particular mode plus the costs of the different modes relative to one another.

In Crane's view, calls for improving connectivity and proximity so as to increase the share of trips by transit, by foot, or on bicycle all fail to take these costs into account. What happens, he asks, if the cost of travel by car falls more rapidly than for walking or biking as the result of such improvements? Trip making by car may increase. Simultaneously, trip making by alternative modes may decrease, stay the same, or increase, all depending on the changes to the relative cost of each mode vis-à-vis that of driving. Crane admits that it is difficult to predict in advance the effects of any design change. The combined effect of any given design will be ambiguous and specific to the combination of elements that make up the built environment in the area. In support of Crane's argument, research has demonstrated that households located in areas with higher connectivity generate more pedestrian and more auto based trips as well. This increase in trip making (also known as trip generation, meaning the number of trips taken) can be explained through the higher utility level provided by a more efficient transportation system. However, the relationship between vehicle and nonmotorized travel is not well understood. That is, it remains an open question as to whether additional vehicle trips result in fewer nonmotorized trips (or vice versa) or whether there is no trade-off between modes. In certain instances, some types of changes will be mode-specific, meaning that the change is specifically geared toward increasing the costs of one mode while decreasing those of others. An example is traffic calming, which is hypothesized to dampen the local demand for automobile trips because it increases the cost of auto trips by increasing the amount of time it takes to traverse a street or neighborhood by car. As a result, traffic calming makes travel by other modes for short trips more attractive, in part because the cost of auto travel is increased relative to alternative modes and in part because the changes that traffic calming introduce to the street often makes travel along those streets more pleasant and safe for walkers and bicyclists (Crane 1999, 1996a, 1996b).

One implication of Crane's argument is the need for urban design solutions that foster lower costs for physical activity in the built environment while maintaining or increasing the cost structure for motorized modes of transportation. For example, many residential subdivisions are physically detached from adjoining retail development (see chapter 8). By retrofitting an area with pathways for nonmotorists, direct connections between the residential development and the retail development could be established for nonmotorists. As a result, the cost of walking and bicycling would fall relative to that of driving because more connectivity has been created for the nonmotorized modes while that for the automobile would remain the same.

A built environment that promotes more walking and biking has a meaningful health benefit regardless of other transportation considerations. Nonetheless, while the decision to walk or bike regardless of the trade-offs between modes is important, the question of mode choice does remain relevant to the discussion. A major reason is due to the possibility that people may have a fixed number of hours that they're willing to invest in travel each day. There is some evidence to suggest that the total amount of time spent traveling, when taking all modes into account, has been relatively constant over the past several decades. This has been referred to as the "law of constant travel time" (Hupkes 1982) and has been estimated to be between one and one and a half hours per day for many people (Schafer and Victor 1997). If people were only willing to spend a certain amount of time each day traveling, then more time spent driving would reduce the amount they'd be willing to travel on foot and by bicycle, and vice versa. This observation still treats travel as involving costs, but differs from the micro-economic model because it both emphasizes time as the key variable and because it focuses on how people allocate their time within a fixed budget instead of on how people weight the relative costs of each type of travel against one another.

A more important point concerns the underlying premises behind micro-economic theory. The theory posits an important question about the effects of the redesign of urban space to improve proximity and connectivity. It is reasonable to assert that people will not substitute walking and bicycling for driving in such environments. This perspective, however, fails to acknowledge that without higher connectivity and proximity in most parts of most American cities, the question of utilitarian walking and biking is an absolute nonstarter in the first place. In many parts of American cities, one cannot even begin to discuss walking and bicycling as serious transportation options without changing development patterns to shorten distances between destinations. Recall from chapter 4 that utilitarian walking and bicycling trips tend to be short. As travel distances increase from a half mile to two and a half miles, the proportion of trips taken on foot declines dramatically. While higher levels of proximity and connectivity may result in more driving trips (although not necessarily more miles driven), such changes to the built environment are fundamental if nonmotorized travel is to have any chance of moving from the margins to the center of urban transportation in the United States. In other countries where distances between destinations are short, and where, not coincidentally, uses are mixed, densities are high, and the transportation infrastructure is multimodal, walking and bicycling are in fact important forms of urban transportation. Shortening distances is a necessary strategy for increasing utilitarian physical activity, but it is not sufficient; other factors, such as urban design variables and transportation system characteristics, are fundamental as well.

Another critique that can be leveled against the micro-economic perspective concerns its singular emphasis upon utility. Micro-economic theory logically requires a focus on individual calculations of loss versus gain, namely, the time and monetary cost involved in travel. Questions involving the user's perception of the spaces in which travel occurs are dismissed almost entirely. The efficient movement of automobile traffic—where efficiency is defined by high average speed and lack of traffic congestion— has long been the standard amongst transportation engineers and many planners for judging the basic soundness of a transportation system. When viewing the world from behind a windshield, the idea that a transportation system should be evaluated according to how quickly and easily one can move from point A to point B makes perfect sense. The point of driving, after all, is to move between destinations at a high rate of speed. It is assumed that the motorist, who exists in a metal and glass cocoon insulated from the surrounding environment, cares little about qualitative issues such as the aesthetics of the roadway and surrounding development. But to the nonmotorist, the external environment has tremendous importance, directly influencing one's perception of the desirability of travel on foot or by bicycle. This is because a walker or bicyclist is much more exposed to external conditions than the motorist. The built environment can be highly pleasant, interesting, and safe or highly unpleasant, uninteresting, and unsafe for the nonmotorist. It is not a stretch to claim that transportation systems and land use patterns that allow for efficient automobile movement are directly at odds with the interests of nonmotorists, because the same environments that promote fast driving are almost always the environments that are unpleasant and unsafe for the walker and bicyclist. All of these issues are discussed at length in the following chapters. For certain, the efficiency of movement within the built environment across each mode is an important consideration to a person who is making a decision about how to get from place to place. However, the important idea is that efficiency cannot, and should not, be viewed as the sole determinant of whether someone will be utilizing nonmotorized means of travel.

Finally, a point must be made about the importance of equity in any debate involving the efficiency of a city's transportation network. As chapter 5 showed, the population should not be treated as a homogenous mass consisting of able-bodied, middle-aged, and relatively affluent people who have the means and ability to drive an automobile. Indeed, for some segments of the population, auto-dependent development is highly inequitable. The micro-economic perspective concentrates on whether people will substitute walking and bicycling for driving and takes it for granted that the answer to this question is ethically neutral, at least with respect to the public policy implications that follow such an analysis—again, the measure by which the system is judged is the efficiency of movement. It does not include questions that might have equal, if not more, surface validity; for example, how transportation systems can be built to serve the needs of everyone or how the built environment can be reorganized to promote public health through walking and bicycling.

RESIDENTIAL SELF-SELECTION

A final problem has to do with the issue of self-selection, which refers to how differences in behavior may be more readily explained by the values of the people being observed than by the phenomenon that supposedly explains the behavior. In terms of the built environment, arguments based upon self-selection assert that any observed differences in behavior in, say, one type of neighborhood versus another type have more to do with the kind of people who choose to live in each type of neighborhood than it does with the attributes of the neighborhoods themselves. Many studies, some of which will be reviewed in the following chapters, find that people walk and bicycle more in neighborhoods that offer higher levels of proximity and connectivity between activities than people who live in the typical suburb. These patterns hold even when the researchers control for the independent influence of wealth and other socioeconomic indicators by choosing, say, two neighborhoods that have the same demographic characteristics but differ in terms of how they were built. To some critics, such findings are suspect because they fail to consider that the people who live in each neighborhood may have different values with respect to relevant variables in the study, for example, how much they value driving versus transit or bicycling. These critics observe that even within similar demographic groups there are widely differing sets of opinions about many types of things that might influence behavior. People who live in dense, mixed-use neighborhoods may choose to live there because they want to be able to walk and, in turn, they may want to walk because of concerns about the negative social and environmental effects of driving. A few studies that have considered the role of values in travel behavior have found that they have a role in directing how much someone drives, walks, or bicycles (e.g., Kitamura, Mokhtarian, and Laidet 1994). There have even been some studies, using data collected from the same households over a couple of years, that have found that people who move from one type of neighborhood to a different type (say, from low to high density) do not automatically change their behavior. Rather, their previous habits remain after moving (Krizek 2000).

As with the micro-economic perspective, the self-selection theory raises a perfectly valid point. It is reasonable to assert that some people value driving more than others, and vice versa in the case of walking and bicycling. It is also reasonable to argue that people who choose to live in higher density, mixed-use, and transit-oriented neighborhoods may have different beliefs with respect to social, political, cultural, and environmental issues—this view rests, to some extent, on basic stereotypes of the suburban versus the urban middle and upper-middle-class resident. The built environment, of course, cannot explain everything. With respect to travel, this has been known to be true for many years, as research has shown that income, family size, age, and other socioeconomic and demographic variables have important influences on travel. As a result, if everyone living in the low-density and single-use suburbs were magically transplanted into high density and mixed-use neighborhoods, travel patterns might change but perhaps not as much as might be expected, at least not initially.

The self-selection theory has, however, a number of weaknesses. Implicit within the self-selection argument is the premise that people are living where they ideally want to live; those who live in the suburbs want to live in low-density, single use suburbs and those who live in more urban or neo-traditional neighborhoods are living where they wish as well. This is the classic market-based formulation that is often employed against those who seek to use instruments of public control—land use planning and public infrastructure investment, primarily—to change prevailing development patterns. The self-selection argument largely fails to consider the possibility that a segment, perhaps even a significant segment, of the population is unable to find suitable housing in a neighborhood that meets their preferences. This argument makes the most sense for people who currently live in contemporary suburban neighborhoods but who may wish to live in a more urban one—because there are so few of the latter, there is a good chance that such neighborhoods are undersupplied with respect to demand. For example, less than one-half of a percent of the Atlanta region consists of land use patterns and transportation system characteristics that are needed to make walking a reasonable travel mode for shopping and other nonwork related activities.[2] Given this type of regional condition, households that have a preference for neighborhoods that are denser, mixed use, and walkable will not be able to express their preferences (Levine 1999). The strength of the self-selection argument, therefore, is weakened if neighborhood supply (meaning the supply of a diverse array of neighborhood types) does not align with preferences.

Long-term demographic shifts in the population have resulted in more households that have an interest in seeing different types of housing and neighborhoods come onto the market. These groups, including households without children and households headed by senior citizens, may have a stronger preference for neo-traditional design attributes than other groups, preferences that are not reflected in the housing market (Myers and Gearin 2001). There is increasing evidence to suggest that there is a gap between supply and demand in the residential marketplace with respect to neo-traditional neighborhoods; one study that compared the housing preferences of Bostonians to Atlantans, for example, found that Atlantans have a smaller range of neighborhoods to choose from than Bostonians, resulting in fewer residents of Atlanta being able to find exactly what they were looking for (Levine et al. 2002). The study had chosen these two cities because of the higher percentage of neo-traditional neighborhoods in the older Boston region compared to the newer Atlanta region, which has grown into a major city only within the last quarter century. There are fewer neo-traditional neighborhoods from which to choose in Atlanta than in Boston. As a result, the authors wrote, Atlanta residents who stated that they would like to live in neo-traditional neighborhoods actually lived in neighborhoods of this type much less often than did Bostonians who had the same preference. The researchers concluded that public land use controls in Atlanta, particularly on the region's periphery, had constrained development in such a way as to limit Atlantans' ability to express their preferences for neo-traditional neighborhoods in the marketplace. There is other evidence to support this particular study's findings. An unrelated community preference survey conducted in Atlanta in 2002 revealed that more than one third of the respondents who stated they live in a single use environment would prefer to live in a mixed-use environment where they could walk to nearby shops and services in their next home.[3]

There is, however, a second and an even more basic weakness in the self-selection model, having to do with the role played by the built environment in shaping thought patterns, expectations, and behavior in that environment. As Kevin Krizek, an academic planner and proponent of the self-selection model, has written, "individual determinants of travel behavior are firmly embedded in cultural and attitudinal approaches to travel" (Krizek 2000, 54). Culture does matter (vague though the concept of culture may be), for it *does* shape attitudes, expectations, and behavior about all sorts of things, travel behavior included. Yet the cultural argument is just as easily employed against the theory of self-selection as it is in favor of the theory. The majority of adult Americans have lived their entire lives in environments that necessitate automobile travel and that make travel by other modes, at least for utilitarian purposes, virtually impossible. It is not an exaggeration to say that the overwhelming majority of development in the United States for the past seventy years has been low density, single use, and auto-oriented, with nearly all of it occurring in the suburbs. One can hardly expect that the attitudes and behavior amongst a good percentage of the suburban population would change immediately and dramatically were one to somehow uproot them and replant them in more highly connected and proximate environments. To make an even more painfully obvious point, one cannot expect that the majority of Americans could envision serious alternatives to the dominant form of development in this country, given the preponderance of the modern suburb that has been stamped out, production-line style, across the nation. Nor, for that matter, can one expect that many know that other people in other wealthy countries, and even some people in this country, have entirely different ways of living and acting within urban space, ways that might be more enjoyable or convenient or healthy. While a minority of the population does seem to understand that serious development alternatives exist or could exist, for the majority the perception of growth and development issues seems to be heavily influenced by the unidimensional nature of the world that Americans inhabit.

Take for example the recent observations made by two analysts of the residential housing market in the United States, Laurie Volk and Todd Zimmerman. According to these analysts, opinion surveys that show unstable and even contradictory results with respect to ideas about development, neighborhood design, and housing (for example, the common finding that many people want larger houses on bigger lots but also want less traffic) "serve to support our contention that Americans are incapable of responding reliably to questions, even unambiguous questions, that depend on an understanding of physical form; many, if not most, Americans lack any frame of reference. The baby boomers in particular, when compared with previous generations, have had as a whole very limited neighborhood experience. The rapidly suburbanizing America in which they grew up [changed] forever many Americans' perception of the characteristics of a 'normal' residential neighborhood"

(Volk and Zimmerman 2001, 678). In other words, the cultural premise that lies behind self-selection theory may itself rest upon a spatial foundation. If, as Winston Churchill once famously said in a speech to the House of Commons, "we shape our buildings, and afterwards our buildings shape us," then much of the force behind the self-selection argument is blunted because the built environment creates cultural attitudes and predispositions as much as the other way around. Admittedly, culture changes slowly, so it is reasonable to believe that alterations to the built environment will change attitudes and behavior across a wide spectrum of the population only over the longer term. Nonetheless, it can be done and, in fact, has been done once already in the history of this country—people used to walk, bike, and take transit in droves before the world was rebuilt to make driving as convenient as possible.

CHAPTER SEVEN

Transportation Systems

Transportation systems can be mapped in terms of the physical infrastructure that carries traffic—streets, rail lines for mass transit, and so on. Alternatively, they can be mapped in terms of the totality of networks for use by each individual mode, such as the bicycle. The former would articulate the transportation system in terms with which everyone is familiar, as a map containing streets, transit lines, and the like. The latter would be more of a conceptual map of a mode-specific network, on which the total amount of infrastructure dedicated to a specific mode would be shown. For example, for pedestrians such a map might contain streets with sidewalks, pathways within city park boundaries, and biking/hiking trails (generally speaking, paved systems designed for use by pedestrians, bicyclists, rollerbladers, etc.). In the following sections, we focus on each of the physical pieces of the various transportation networks that are relevant to travel by pedestrians and bicyclists.

Street Networks

Streets, and the spaces immediately adjacent to streets such as sidewalks, form the most ubiquitous type of transportation network. Their importance for travel by all modes cannot be overstated, for they connect nearly every destination to one another within cities. No other type of transportation system can begin to approach the comprehensiveness of a city's street network. Additionally, because streets are so ubiquitous, they are an important dimension of the urban fabric in their own right, contributing to a city's sense of place, or lack thereof. This chapter is focused on the ways in which streets connect places to one another; street design is addressed in detail in chapter 9.

Street networks influence trip route and mode choice through the ways in which trip origins and destinations are connected. Networks can be rated as either high in connectivity, where there are a large number of blocks and intersections per some unit of area, or low in connectivity, where there are fewer blocks and intersections over the same area. In its simplest formulation, the greater the number of intersections over a given area, the more direct a route is likely to be from any randomly selected destination to any other. More intersections make it easier to trace a relatively direct line along the street network between two destinations. Because the network has streets that cross at frequent intervals, a person situated along any given street segment will not have to travel far in order to turn in the direction of his or her intended destination. Such a system minimizes the disparity between the crow-fly distance between two points and the distance one must travel on the ground between those same points. For the nonmotorist, minimizing this disparity is critical, as longer trips are rarely taken on foot or by bicycle, for obvious reasons.

This concept is illustrated in figure 7-1. The image on the left represents the high-connectivity network. Here, because there are many connections between various points, the traveler will be more likely to have both a more direct route and more route options between any two points A and B. In contrast, the low-connectivity network, represented by the image on the right, forces people to travel a greater distance over the street network in order to reach their destination. In this hypothetical example, although the crow-fly distance is the same as in the left-hand diagram, a person would have to travel a far greater distance because the street network contains very few connections between these destinations.

There are three general types of street networks. These are the organic, grid, and hierarchical street networks. The typology used here follows that of architectural historian A. E. J. Morris, who contrasts organic forms of urban growth with planned forms. Morris defines organic growth as "the natural, unplanned process whereby an urban settlement evolves from a village origin" without planned intervention. In contrast, planned urban form "is the result of predetermined intention" by a local government and/or professional planners, engineers, and architects (Morris 1994, 8, 10). Applied to street net-

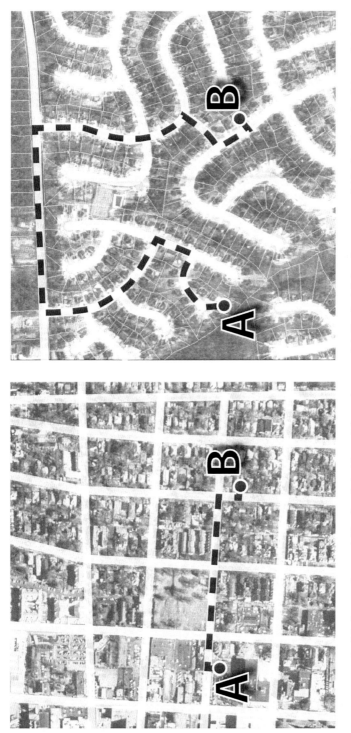

FIGURE 7-1. Aerial photos of two neighborhoods in Metro Atlanta (same scale). On the left is a downtown neighborhood, on the right a suburban neighborhood. The distance one would have to travel along the street network to get from two equidistant points (A and B) is much less along the downtown network (left) versus along the suburban network (right).

works, the grid and hierarchical networks fall into the planned growth category. Conversely, as the name implies, organic networks result from gradual, unplanned changes made to street systems over many centuries. These networks, or remnants of networks, can be found in the oldest parts of many European, Asian, and African cities. While there are many forms of organic networks, typically such networks were bounded by the city's defensive wall with an important civic, religious, or political structure (a marketplace, church or temple, or town hall) at the center. Streets radiated in all directions, resulting in a crazy-quilt pattern (figure 7-2). Although streets in organic networks are narrow and winding, most often the multiple interconnected streets form small, tight blocks, allowing for short distances and multiple linkages between destinations. In some ancient Middle Eastern cities, the pattern evolved to resemble a modern cul-de-sac arrangement. In all layouts, however, walking was a very efficient mode of transportation due to the short distances between trip destinations—an unsurprising result given that humans and animals provided the only means of transportation during the centuries in which these networks evolved. The limitation of the organic street network, of course, is that it doesn't exist at all outside of the oldest sections of the oldest cities—it exists in very old places precisely because it had to be built piecemeal over decades or even centuries. Planned networks, whether grids, variations on the grid, or hierarchical and discontinuous networks, are the norm in virtually all sections of all contemporary cities, and will remain so into the future.

The archetype of the planned high connectivity network is the grid pattern (figure 7-3). The gridiron is a simple system of two sets of parallel streets crossing at right angles to form square or rectangular blocks. The pure grid system has streets that are nonhierarchical, that is, there is no differentiation of streets by either traffic volume or street width. There are variations on the pure grid pattern, of course, resulting in modified grids that contain diagonals, have irregularly sized blocks, or have some differentiation by street width—one example is the street network created by Pierre L'Enfant for Washington, D.C., containing multiple diagonals overlaid against a traditional grid (figure 7-4). (L'Enfant intended that his street network would create grandeur and a sense of order for the nation's capital. His axial approach allowed monuments and significant public buildings to be located at the intersections of major corridors, creating a sight line leading to a focal point

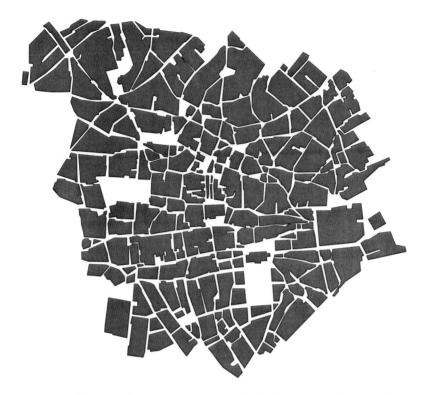

FIGURE 7-2. Diagram of an organic street network, in this case the oldest part of Seville, Spain. This part of the city is only about a mile from east to west, yet there are dozens of streets, most of which are narrow and winding.

on the horizon. One can hardly find a location within D.C. that does not offer, or is not adjacent to, a sight line of interest.)

The gridiron is a very old form of street network configuration. Gridlike street patterns have been found in the remains of many ancient settlements, including Egyptian, Indian, and Greek cities. The grid was the basis of Roman urban planning, providing the earliest street networks for many towns that the Romans established across Europe and North Africa (in many of these cities, the original grid would be gradually supplanted and replaced by organic networks during the intervening centuries between the collapse of the Roman Empire and the late Middle Ages) (Morris 1994). The grid found much appeal in later centuries as well. In the early history of the United States, many cities were laid out using the grid. Grids provided coherence to rapidly growing cities along the east coast, simplifying real

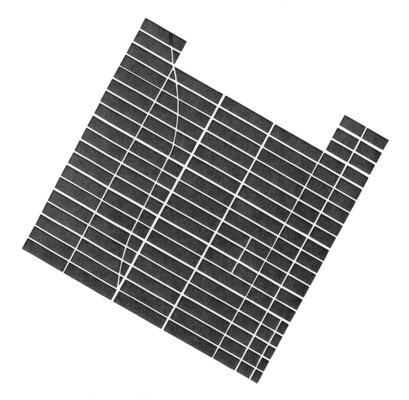

FIGURE 7-3. Diagram of a "pure" grid street network—lower Manhattan from 43rd Street to Central Park. Only Broadway's curvilinear shape interrupts the grid's regularity.

estate transactions (standardized, geometrical block sizes made land speculation far easier) and making transportation within cities more efficient (Moudon and Untermann 1987). Grids were established in many early American cities, including New York, Philadelphia, Washington, and Savannah. As the nation expanded westward, so too did the grid design, finding its way into the street systems of major midwestern and western cities such as Chicago and San Francisco.

The third type of street network, the hierarchical pattern, has been widely employed in the United States since the middle of the twentieth century (figure 7-5). While there are examples of hierarchical street networks that arose organically in ancient cities, today's networks have been created as one solution to the problems imposed by the automobile on the urban landscape. Hierarchical networks reject the principles upon which the grid was founded.

In this type of system, which has a number of variations, streets are deliberately ordered into a hierarchy that is based upon traffic movement. At the top of the hierarchy are major arterial roads, which are designed primarily for high-volume automobile traffic and often feature no amenities for bicyclists or pedestrians. At the bottom of the hierarchy are local residential streets, which are designed to ensure a low volume of through traffic by automobiles. Residential streets are, in effect, privatized in this system as they become the domain of neighborhood residents only. These streets loop back on themselves or terminate as cul-de-sacs. Most often, a residential subdivision consists of a number of such streets, which join at a single point along the arterial system, disgorging the total amount of traffic that the subdivision generates at that point. Such networks contain a low number of blocks and intersections per unit of area. The significance for physical activity is that such networks increase trip lengths and decrease the number of choices available to the traveler, via a reduction in the number of available routes as well as the number of practical modes (Frank 2000; Southworth and Owens 1993).

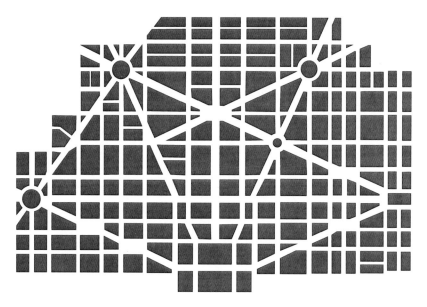

FIGURE 7-4. Diagram of a "modified" grid street network—Washington, D.C. The White House grounds are at the bottom of the diagram. Pierre L'Enfant, Washington's planner, overlaid diagonals against a grid network in order to give the city a monumental flourish.

Discontent with certain aspects of the grid layout in the United States began in the nineteenth century. As was discussed in detail in chapter 2, at the end of that century reformers were associating the grid with many of the social and economic ills that plagued American cities. In their view, the monotony of the grid gave little attention to the open space needs of urban populations, fostered substandard housing, and allowed too little light and fresh air into the city. The judgment against the grid extended as well to aesthetic considerations: the grid stamped a rigid geometry onto undulating landscapes (Wolfe 1987). Clarence Stein, of Radburn fame, hated the grid, believing that it stifled creative neighborhood designs that would produce more light, green space, and better housing for residents (Stein 1957). He built into the Radburn layout a street network that was deliberately intended to break up the grid, introducing the basic hierarchical pattern that is now the template for virtually all new development in the United States. Neighborhoods would be composed primarily of cul-de-sacs for residential use only, with the entire neighborhood attached to one or two "connectors" that would in turn feed the "arterials" that were designed exclusively for moving traffic across the city. Clarence Perry, who, as discussed previously, formulated ideas that were central to the design of Radburn's network, felt the same with respect to the design of his Neighborhood Planning Units. His goal was to make automobile trips across his neighborhoods as difficult as possible, while making such trips on the edges of the neighborhood as simple and as fast as possible. To do this, Perry proposed making interior streets "inconvenient and forbidding for vehicles having no destination within the neighborhood confines" (Perry 1939, 56). In contrast, the streets on the edge would be designed for fast vehicle travel; through traffic would thereby be routed onto the connectors and arterials that were placed at the edges of the neighborhood.[1] These were watershed ideas in the history of American planning. In 1936, the newly formed Federal Housing Administration (FHA) issued a bulletin recommending the adoption of these principles in subdivision design. The FHA would come to wield enormous influence during the postwar period, when its subdivision design recommendations became the standard for suburban development in the United States, resulting in the institutionalization of the hierarchical street network across the country (Southworth and Ben-Joseph 2003, 1995).

The condemnation of the grid in the United States was at least in part the

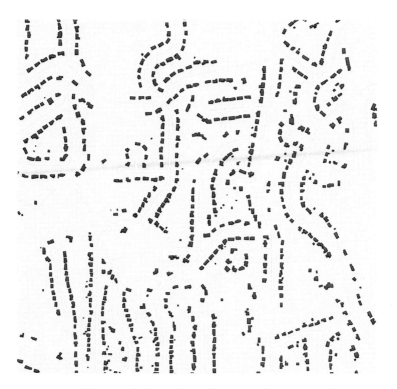

FIGURE 7-5. Diagram of a hierarchical, disconnected street network in suburban Atlanta.

result of the fact that the grid happened to be the prevailing street pattern during a period in history of extreme disenchantment with all aspects of the city. There is no inherent reason why grids cannot provide the same health benefits as more discontinuous street networks. Napoleon III's reconstruction of Paris during the mid-nineteenth century, for example, removed much of the city's narrow, winding street infrastructure and replaced it with its current gridlike network of wide boulevards. While this reconstruction was intended to improve connectivity between major destinations within the city, another purpose was to improve public health. The broad boulevards would, so Georges-Eugene Haussmann, chief architect of the reconstruction, believed, introduce more light and air into the city, thereby contributing to the health of the city's residents (Saalman 1971). American planners of the early to mid-twentieth century had different opinions, however, about the virtues of the grid. Their views can be interpreted within the context of a larger movement that de-emphasized the city altogether. Solutions to urban problems were to be resolved primarily through the creation of new settlements within the vast countryside of the United States. In their view, the isolated and self-contained neighborhoods of new suburban communities promised to deliver to Americans, or at least those who could afford them, the benefits of the city without any of its drawbacks. Influential American planners of the early twentieth century subscribed to the belief that sufficient light, fresh air, and greenspace could not be provided using the traditional grid design. Self-contained, neighborhood-based planning required the creation of alternatives to the grid (Wolfe 1987).

During the immediate postwar period, professional groups and government agencies advocated the use of these principles, which became widely incorporated into the design of new suburbs. Illustrative is a 1948 report issued by the American Public Health Association's Committee on the Hygiene of Housing. The committee had long been active in generating reports connecting housing to health; prior to the war, it had released two reports on residential construction principles for health. The report issued in 1948 focused on neighborhood planning and included a section on traffic circulation systems. The committee advocated a hierarchical street classification scheme, stating bluntly that neighborhoods should be as disconnected as possible. "To discourage through traffic through the neighborhood," it recommended, "streets should be so laid out that no streets within the neighborhood can be used as a short cut between two points outside it. . . . This may be accomplished by loop or dead-end streets" (American Public Health Administration 1948). In each successive decade after the war, planners and developers have greatly increased the level of hierarchy, curvilinearity, and disconnectedness of the street network. Over this time period, street networks have transitioned from the rigidly geometric to the extremely disconnected and curvilinear. The result has been that postwar communities, in contrast to those built in earlier decades, have street networks containing fewer intersections, blocks, and external access points as well as a greater number of loops and cul-de-sacs on interior streets (Southworth and Owens 1993).

The disconnected network has come under a good deal of scrutiny over the past decade, most of which has centered around the connectivity problems

created by such designs as well as the basic dangers associated with nonmotorized travel along arterial roads. While hierarchical networks can offer
internal havens from through traffic, and offer places where children can play
in the streets, they reduce connectivity and impede functional access between
complementary land uses. With respect to the latter problem, hierarchical
networks introduce major problems for anyone attempting a trip on foot or
by bicycle to a destination outside of one's neighborhood. Arterials make
travel on foot or by bicycle dangerous and impractical across neighborhood
boundaries (Untermann 1987). To some extent, of course, this is as intended:
such networks were originally meant in part to create physical barriers for
movement on foot across and between neighborhoods. Unfortunately, however, subdivisions built during the second half of the twentieth century rarely
contained the pedestrian-friendly components that Clarence Perry and others advocated, such as schools and retail destinations, parks, and even some
mixing of uses and housing types. Postwar designs have retained only the
basic street network concept while neglecting to include highly localized
amenities such as light retail, elementary schools, and small parks, making it
impossible for people to reach nonresidential destinations within their
neighborhoods.

Specialized Networks for Nonmotorists

The second type of transportation network consists of those facilities that are
both off-street (i.e., not a part of either the street surface or the area immediately adjacent to the street) and that are dedicated to the nonmotorized
modes of transportation and some forms of recreational physical activity.
These networks include specialized bicycle facilities, shared facilities that
accommodate multiple uses (such as trails for bicyclists, joggers, and
rollerbladers that utilize abandoned railway lines), and pedestrian- and/or
bicyclist-only paths that are designed to provide linkages for users of these
modes (but not for other modes) between in-town destinations. Specialized
networks for bicyclists have been constructed in many European cities and
towns, where they serve to provide a practical means of getting around within
cities (photos 7-1 and 7-2). Such networks have been created most aggres-
sively in the Netherlands. As a central goal of Dutch transportation policy is

to make alternative modes of travel easy, safe, and accessible, authorities have for years invested heavily in facilities geared toward these modes. Their systems consist of more than just lengthy networks of separated bike paths and bike lanes along streets; they also include bus lanes that can be used by bicycles but not cars, streets that give bicyclists right-of-way priority over cars, and a series of ingenious street design treatments that provide short-cuts for bicyclists but not for motorists. The result is a fine-grained network of bike-specific facilities that connect practical destinations within Dutch cities, making the bicycle a practical means of traveling within their urbanized areas. These networks play a central role in giving the Netherlands one of the highest mode shares for bicycling in the world. Other northern European countries—notably Germany—have instituted similar policies, resulting in impressive gains in trips made by bicycle in that country over the last twenty years (Pucher and Dijkstra 2000).

Off-street facilities for bicyclists in the United States are both much more limited than in Europe and tend to be oriented toward recreational bicycling. Some American cities (or, more accurately, university towns such as Davis, California, and Boulder, Colorado) have extensive bicycling facilities. There have been some gains at the national level as well. Much has been made, for instance, of the federal government's turnaround in funding for bicycling facilities during the 1990s under the Intermodal Surface Transportation Act (ISTEA). This legislation significantly increased the amount of federal funds available for bicycle projects and became the source of funding for a large number of off-street bicycle facilities. The Rails-to-Trails Conservancy, a group that advocates the conversion of recreational bicycle and pedestrian systems from converted railroad lines, estimates that in 2002 there were some 1,100 trails and 11,000 trail miles in the United States.[2] These trails do not represent the entirety of the nation's off-street bicycle and pedestrian network, but they do comprise a significant portion of the dedicated off-street infrastructure for these modes. Yet the disparity between these types of facilities and the sheer size of the street network in the United States (there are some four million miles of streets, roads, and highways in the U.S.) illustrates the gap between the two types of transportation networks (U.S. Department of Transportation 2001). Given that most off-street bicycling trails are in rural areas and are designed with recreational exercise in mind, these facilities

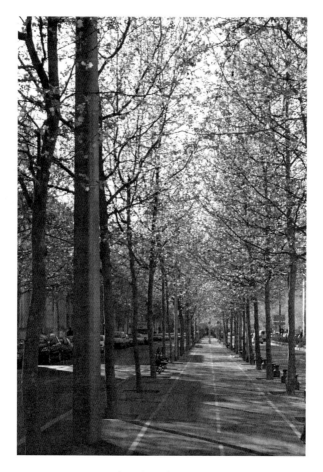

PHOTO 7-1. In-town bicycle path in Montpelier, France, built
into the street median.

cannot, in most instances, be used for day-to-day intra-urban travel (Pucher,
Komanoff, and Schimek 1999).

Within the community of bicycling advocates in the United States, there is
considerable controversy surrounding the question of whether infrastruc-
tural investments should be made in separated (off-street) bicycle facilities or
on-street facilities. Some advocates, led most notably by John Forester, contend that as bicycling is more appropriate on existing streets rather than on
separated facilities, public and private resources should be devoted to the creation of on-street facilities and to educating drivers and bicyclists about the

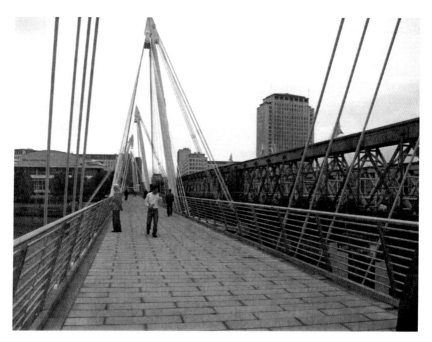

PHOTO 7-2. Hungerford cable stayed pedestrian bridge, London, over the Thames. Investment in exclusively nonmotorized infrastructure provides linkages between destinations for these modes.

rights and responsibilities of bicyclists. They argue that bicyclists should be treated similarly to motorists, with the same rights to the use of the street as well as the same responsibilities with respect to following traffic laws. Much of Forester's argument rests upon the assertion that separated facilities are actually more dangerous to bicyclists than riding on-street, a claim that has drawn much criticism (Forester 2001; Pucher 2001). Others in this camp also claim that off-street facilities serve to weaken the legitimacy of bicyclists as users of the street. As they see it, the creation of such networks will further marginalize bicyclists by reinforcing the idea that the street is not a place for bicycling. Conversely, those who want to see the creation of specialized off-street systems assert that these systems are safer and, theoretically, can be very convenient if they connect practical destinations. Further, they contend that the creation of more and better off-street systems does not negate the need to redesign streets to be bicycle-friendly. They hold that while efforts should be made to redesign streets to make them safer and more attractive to bicyclists, the facts, especially from cities in Europe that have heavily invested in off-street bicycling networks, demonstrate that such systems can be an important component of a bicycling-friendly transportation system (Pucher 2001).

Transit Systems

Finally, a word or two must be said about the relationships between transit and nonmotorized forms of transportation. Transit and walking are considered to be two modes that are ideally suited to one another, although bicycling can also be made to work well with transit.[3] The reason, of course, is the nature of transit service: one needs to both get to the transit stop at the beginning and get to destinations of interest to the transit rider at the end. This requires that at least one of the segments of the journey be on foot. The beginning part of the journey, from home or some other place to the transit stop, can, of course, be made by car. This is often the case in rail systems that were built to fulfill the needs of suburban commuters who want to get into the central business district. In such systems, transit stops that are built in the suburbs are surrounded by parking lots in order to attract commuters (photo 7-3). These stations, essentially, have no other use because the surrounding lots separate the station from nearby development, making it too far away to allow someone to walk to the station from home or to allow someone to walk from the station to, say, a shopping center. At the other end of the transit journey, on the other hand, the rider has no choice but to finish his or her trip on foot. In the case of the commuter, most often this means getting off the transit system downtown and walking to work.

In contrast, when transit is integrated into the built environment—on both ends of the transit journey—it allows the rider to abandon his or her dependency on the car altogether (photo 7-4). This is most pronounced in areas that are compactly built and pedestrian friendly, qualities that used to be widely found in those areas of American cities that were serviced by trolleys. The design of places to encourage the transit/walking combination is the central idea behind the concept of "transit-oriented development" (TOD), a phrase coined by Peter Calthorpe. Pedestrians, Calthorpe argued, "like transit to extend their range of destinations. These needs can be satisfied in both high-density urban centers and small mixed-use towns, but not in sprawling,

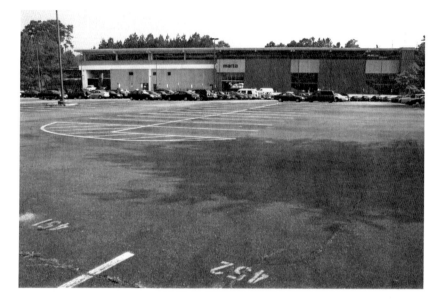

PHOTO 7-3. Transit station, Atlanta, Georgia. Many suburban transit stations are designed with the commuter in mind and are therefore surrounded by huge parking lots, breaking the natural link between transit and walking by isolating the station from adjacent development.

unplanned suburbs." The TOD concept, therefore, "is simple: moderate and high-density housing, along with complementary public uses, jobs, retail and services, are concentrated in mixed-use developments at strategic points along the regional transit system" (Calthorpe 1993, 27–8, 41).

Evidence

Different transportation systems have an influence on how people travel, including travel on foot or by bicycle. Some research has focused exclusively or primarily on transportation system characteristics, despite the problem involving spatial co-variance that was discussed in the last chapter. Results from several studies will be discussed in this section by way of illustration. A number have employed quasi-experimental, neighborhood-based research designs. One, by Moudon et al. (Moudon et al. 1997) selected for analysis twelve neighborhoods in the Puget Sound area. They controlled for density, mixture of uses, and regional location to isolate the effect of street network connectivity and the safety of pedestrian facilities on pedestrian travel within these neighborhoods. Half of the neighborhoods had grid street networks and high-quality pedestrian facilities (safe rights-of-way, continuous sidewalk networks, direct pedestrian routes between residential and commercial development, and so forth). The other half had disconnected street networks and substandard pedestrian facilities and amenities. All twelve neighborhoods contained small- and medium-sized commercial centers and were surrounded by medium-density residential development. The six neighborhoods with greater connectivity and better facilities (defined as "urban") generated higher pedestrian traffic volumes than those with poorer levels of connectivity and poorer facilities (defined as "suburban"), defined in terms of the number of pedestrians that passed by an observation point within the neighborhood per hour (table 7-1).

Other studies have attempted to assess how specialized bicycle and pedes-

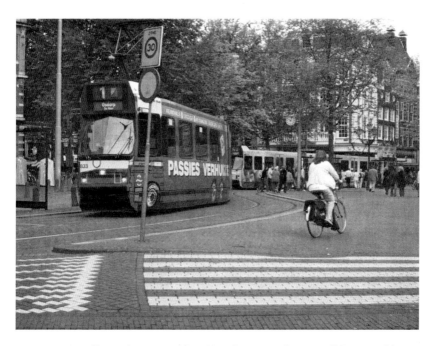

PHOTO 7-4. Trolley station, Amsterdam. Transit systems that are well integrated into existing development make travel on foot much easier because they provide direct access to destinations. They also enhance the quality of the surrounding environment, thereby contributing to a more pleasant walking experience.

TABLE 7-1
*Summary of site design measures and pedestrian volumes: Averages for urban
and suburban sites, Seattle, Washington*

	Urban sites (U)	Suburban sites (S)	U:S ratio
Block size (ha)*	1.1	12.8	1:12.2
Street system length (km)	48.0	15.9	1:0.33
Sidewalk system length (km)	60.5	12.6	1:0.21
Sidewalk system completeness	.97	.55	1:0.57
Population density (people/ha)	34.3	31.5	1:0.92
Population	6,684	6,308	1:0.93
Pedestrians/hour/1,000 residents	38	12	1:0.33
Pedestrians/hour	217	68	1:0.30

*202.5 hectares = 500 acres.

SOURCE: Anne Moudon, Paul Hess, Mary Snyder, Kiril Stanilov, "Effects of site design on pedestrian travel in mixed-use, medium-density environments." Reproduced with permission of the Transportation Research Board. In *Transportation Research Record* 1578, Transportaton Research Board, National Research Council, Washington, D.C., 1997, 48–55.

trian networks influence walking and bicycling. One, of NPTS data from eighteen American cities (Nelson and Allen 1997), attempted to assess the extent to which bicycle networks influenced commuting by bicycle. The authors examined one independent variable (number of bicycle pathway miles per 100,000 residents) and four control variables (terrain characteristics, number of rain days per year, mean high temperature, and percentage of college students) on the percent of commuters using bicycles. The results showed that only bicycle pathway miles, percent of college students, and number of rain days were significantly related to commuting by bicycle. The authors believed that the form of the network—whether the network connects residential areas to employment destinations or is designed for recreational use only (as is the case with most rail-trails)—is likely to be as important as the amount of network mileage in determining commuting behavior.

Far more common are studies of networks within a single city or comparative studies of such networks across cities. For example, one review of the experience of the city of Delft in the Netherlands (Hartman 1993) examined the effect that a new bicycle network had on bicycling and driving over time. Beginning in the late 1970s, the city began the construction of an extensive bicycle network, consisting of several kilometers of paths and lanes, several bicycle-only tunnels and bridges within the city, and the alteration of existing city streets to enhance bicycle mobility and restrict automobile use. The author conducted a before-and-after analysis of two areas of the city, one where changes were made (the study area) and one, the control area, where none were made. In the control area, motor vehicle use increased by 10 percent, with the data suggesting that the increase came at the expense of public transport. In the study area, bicycle usage increased by 6 to 8 percent, with an equal decline in auto use.

Another example of how successful nonmotorized networks can be in inducing walking and bicycling is provided by a study from Germany (Hülsmann 1993). In the 1980s, two cities, Rosenheim and Detmold, created bicycling networks in areas of the city where there had previously been no such infrastructure. The cities created separated bicycle routes and lanes, installed bicycle rental facilities, posted route signs for bicyclists, and instituted bicycle safety and public relations campaigns. In Rosenheim, bicycle traffic increased by 13 percent between 1981 and 1986, with a rise in mode share from 23 percent of all trips to 26 percent of all trips. In contrast, driving did not increase, despite the fact that more people owned cars in 1986 than 1981. This specific finding is consistent with trends in Germany overall. Between the 1970s and 1990s, German municipalities created aggressive public policies to encourage bicycling and discourage automobile use. Cities created extensive bicycle networks, traffic calming schemes, and bike rental facilities in public spaces (town squares, rail depots), and subsidized bicycle travel in a variety of ways. Simultaneously, auto use was discouraged through restricting the supply of parking in downtown areas, prohibiting new roadway construction, and severely restricting vehicle speed limits on many streets. The result was substantial increases in the mode share for bicycles, with an average increase of 50 percent for all urban areas in the western part of Germany over this period (Pucher 1997).

Conclusion

This chapter has identified a variety of ways that transportation investments influence a person's ability to walk and bike in urban areas. Transportation networks shape how people can move about in the built environment, through their influence on the level of access to a range of activities or destinations as well as the amount of mobility (a measure of the ability to move through space). Both the level of accessibility and the level of mobility are a function of the shape and design of a given modal network, but perhaps more importantly the linkages between modes. Transit and nonmotorized forms of transportation can work synergistically. The linkages between these regional (transit) and local (pedestrian and bicycle) transportation systems need to be carefully planned and designed. The provision of bike racks on buses or the emplacement of attractive sidewalk systems between transit stations and adjacent residential and commercial uses will improve the range of choices and increase the drawing power of these modes. Improving the design of inter-modal connections significantly impacts the convenience and attractiveness of alternative transportation options. A critical component of transportation systems planning and design must, therefore, be focused on intermodal terminals. Places such as airports, train stations and transit stops need to be designed to enable quick and convenient access between various legs of a journey in order for alternative modes to become competitive with the automobile.

Approaches to developing transportation networks have changed dramatically over the past century as society has moved from an urban model built upon walking and transit to one designed to facilitate the movement of vehicles. It is no secret that transportation systems in the United States are primarily designed to accommodate the car, often at the direct expense of the pedestrian, cyclist, and transit patron. Behavior in the built environment, including travel behavior as well as physical activity patterns, is not solely a function of transportation networks, however. Land use patterns and urban design characteristics also play a large part in determining behavior. When certain types of land use patterns and urban design characteristics are coupled with certain types of transportation networks, moreover, the effect on walking, bicycling, and other forms of physical activity can be enormous.

CHAPTER EIGHT

Land Use Patterns

L and use patterns represent the arrangement of structures and other features within the built environment. This arrangement of features—of buildings, parks, and so on—determines the degree of proximity between trip origins and destinations. As defined in chapter 6, proximity refers to the closeness of destinations in the environment, regardless of how well or poorly transportation systems connect them. It is possible to have destinations that are proximate but poorly connected, as in the common case of a shopping center bordering a residential subdivision where a wall has been inserted in between them (photo 8-1). Conversely, destinations can be well connected but not proximate. Unfortunately, in most suburban and exurban areas of American cities, destinations are often neither well connected nor proximate.

Two urban form variables will be analyzed in this section. First, the *density* of population and employment over a given spatial area is one of the most widely used indicators of urban form for scholars interested in understanding travel patterns. Density is a measure of compactness. The relationship between density and travel behavior is seemingly uncomplicated and intuitive. Higher density levels (greater compactness), it is reasoned, affect travel behavior by locating activities closer together, reducing the need to use a vehicle and increasing mode choice options. Activities located closer together increase the attractiveness of bicycling and walking, as well as providing the "mass" of population that is necessary for transit to be viable. In reducing distances between destinations, higher density levels also theoretically serve to

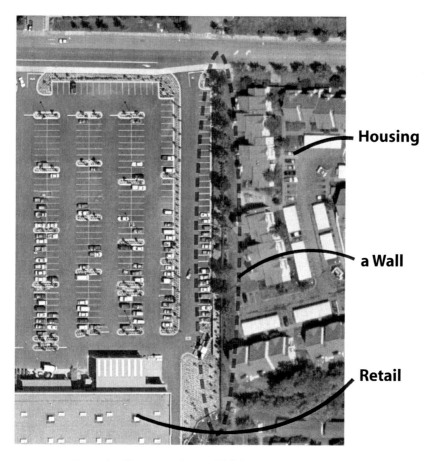

Housing

a Wall

Retail

PHOTO 8-1. Example of how areas that are high in proximity can be low in connectivity. Here, a subdivision and shopping center are located next door to each other, but are separated by a wall.

increase the proximity between facilities that can be used for recreational exercise, such as parks and residential areas.

The second, *land use mix*, also defined in chapter 6, refers to the composition of uses within a geographic area. Most new areas of a city built since the middle of the twentieth century are zoned as single use, with the area contained within them dedicated exclusively to residential, commercial, or industrial uses. As the name implies, areas that are mixed use have a combination of uses within their boundaries. The term "mixed use" is a descriptor for the built environment at different spatial levels, from areas as small as a single building or as large as a neighborhood, a part of a region, or even an entire city. Most frequently, the concept is measured somewhere between the smallest unit (the building) and the largest (the entire city or region). Like density, land use mixing increases the proximity between any two destinations. Ideally, complementary uses including residential, retail, entertainment, recreational, and employment are intermixed over small areas requiring minimum travel distances between activities. The mixing or separation of uses defines how far one needs to travel between different types of destinations. In single-use areas, residential subdivisions are often far from office centers or shopping destinations.

Density

Density, as it is conceived and used here, is a measure of urban form that is meant to convey objective information about how compactly built a place is. Density, it will be recalled, is regarded as an important phenomenon because higher densities have the effect of reducing distances (increasing proximity). The relationship between density and physical activity is often regarded as being axiomatic: higher density levels will produce more walking and biking because distances are shortened. The shortening of distances between destinations is widely believed to increase the odds that a person will shift from driving toward walking, bicycling, and transit use (Apogee 1998).[1] This basic understanding, that density is intimately related to travel behavior, including nonmotorized travel, has long placed the concept at the center of transportation planning studies.

Yet while density has much surface appeal because its relationship to travel appears to be so straightforward, upon closer examination the concept begins to become a good bit more complicated. This begins at the most foundational level. What, exactly, is meant by density, the density of *what?* Most transportation planners rely upon one of several population-based measures to provide an indicator of how compactly built a place is. These measures are used because of the ease with which such data can be found or generated—Census data, for example, is available for all metropolitan regions and is updated every ten years. Therefore, density is almost always measured in terms of the number of people, households, or employees over a given area such as a square mile or kilometer (Dunphy and Fisher 1994). There are many variations, including: household density (the total number of households per a given area of land), residential density (the total number of residents per area), net residential density (total residents per the amount of residential land in an area), and employment density (number of employees per land area, a measure of the intensity of commercial development found in that area) (Frank, Stone, and Bachman 2000).

Reliance on population density is usually motivated by two core beliefs with respect to transportation issues. First, higher population densities make transit more viable, because high concentrations of people provide the ridership that transit needs to be financially feasible. Again, transit stations that are placed in high-density areas should be more successful at attracting riders because the station will be within walking distance of a greater number of people (Parsons Brinckerhoff 1996). But the second belief with respect to population density and travel is more important—higher population densities are believed to translate into shorter on-the-ground distances within the area being studied. The oft-unstated, yet reasonable, assumption is that high population densities are correlated with high concentrations of so-called trip ends in that area, where, as the name implies, a trip end is the beginning or end point of a trip. When the term *density* is employed in discussions concerning transportation issues, much of the concern really has to do with this concentration of trip ends. The implicit belief is that an area that is low in population density has a low concentration of trip ends because there are only a few possible trip origins and destinations contained within that area. In contrast, an area that is high in population density is thought to have a high concentration of trip ends because there are many origins and destinations contained within the area. The premise is that a high concentration of trip ends will produce shorter trip lengths by both shortening the distance one needs to travel between any two points and by reducing the frequency of travel outside of the area in question (by increasing the number and, presumably, type of destinations within the area).

But density is rarely measured in terms of the concentration of trip ends. Obviously, travel behavior is the phenomenon that planners are attempting to model, predict, and explain. The attributes of the built environment—of a city or a suburb or a region—constitute one set of variables that planners use to predict travel behavior. So, the ideal measure of density would be one that closely tracks the concentration of trip ends and yet forms a part of the built environment itself. One such measure might be the density of possible destinations that a person could travel from and to—businesses, post offices, parks, houses, apartments, and so on. A destination isn't necessarily the same thing as a structure, for some destinations aren't structures while some structures contain multiple destinations (think of an office building that houses multiple firms or a building that contains multiple shops). Yet it would be difficult if not impossible to create a measure using destinations to which, and from which, people can travel, especially over a large area such as an entire region. This is because of the huge number of destinations as well as the enormous practical problems of how to generate a list of destinations and obtain data on the precise location and type of destinations that are scattered over a large area. All of this means that population-based density measures will likely remain the standard definition of density for some time to come, with the assumption being that high population densities correlate with shorter on-the-ground distances and vice versa for areas with low population densities.

Another conceptual problem has to do with the definition of high and low density levels. There is little consensus among planners regarding how to classify different densities into "high," "medium," and "low" categories. Different countries have different cultural standards regarding what are considered high and low densities, especially with respect to population density but also with respect to related definitions, such as the density of structures in a city. Naturally enough, planners usually follow their own country's accepted norms when applying numbers to these terms. In countries with lots of people concentrated over a small area, such as Israel or the Netherlands, the numbers attached to high, medium, and even low population densities are higher than in other countries (Churchman 1999). Applied to the American context, these levels are absurdly high; low densities in these countries would in many cases be at the upper end of the American density scale. This basic problem extends to differences at the subnational level as well. In the United States, such definitions can vary widely depending on the metropolitan context— between different regions as well as within regions themselves (Knack 2002).

Finally, it is important to distinguish density from a related concept, crowding. Jane Jacobs, the eminent architectural and planning critic, wrote in her 1961 classic *The Death and Life of Great American Cities* that the two terms should not be confused, even though they routinely are. She distinguished between high densities, defined as a large numbers of dwellings per unit of space, and overcrowding, defined as too many people in a dwelling. Earlier generations of planners, she observed, could not distinguish between these two different ideas when they saw slums that were overcrowded as well as overbuilt. "They hated both equally," Jacobs wrote, "and coupled them like ham and eggs, so that to this day housers and planners pop out the phrase as if it were one word, 'highdensityandovercrowding'" (Jacobs 1993, 268). Jacobs's delicious treatment of the subject highlights a long-standing bias within the American psyche against high densities (Americans, so the joke goes, hate two things: sprawl and density). Her observations about crowding may explain part of the reason why many Americans have such a viscerally negative reaction to high densities, in particular reactions to any proposal that involves increasing densities within already built-up areas. Although high structural densities do not necessarily produce overcrowding (Jacobs observed that wealthy urban residents often live in areas of extremely high structural density, yet the number of residents per room is very low; even today, some of the most affluent neighborhoods in the United States contain extremely high structural densities—think of the wealth that is concentrated in Manhattan or the city of San Francisco), Americans often seem to believe that the two go hand in hand. While density is not a subjective measure of how crowded an area appears to be (here the term *crowded* is used more broadly than used by Jacobs, to mean public crowding—crowding on the street, in parks, in stores, etc.), it is assigned such a meaning by many people (Rapoport 1982). The conflation of density with crowding underscores a need to address how urban form shapes perceptions. Different environments can produce markedly different reactions to similar density levels (Knack 2002). The next chapter on urban design addresses some of these issues, including the importance of the social dimensions of public spaces.

Mixed-Use Development

The phrase "mixed-use development" is, like density, an intuitive term describing the co-location of multiple uses over the same area. It is distinguishable from its logical opposite, "single-use development," which describes the dominant form of development in the United States wherein uses are kept apart from one another. The hypothesized relationship between mixed-use development and physical activity is parallel to that between density and physical activity: the mixing of uses decreases distances between destinations, while separating uses increases those distances. As distance is an important barrier to nonmotorized travel, mixing uses is believed to be an important strategy for increasing travel on foot or by bicycle. The intermixing of uses, particularly retail and commercial uses with residential uses, is a characteristic of older neighborhoods, those designed in the nineteenth and early twentieth centuries (Southworth 1997; Corbett and Velasquez 1994).

Theoretically, mixed-use development could mean the mixing of all types of uses in a single geographic space—commercial, industrial, residential, retail, civic, and entertainment. The phrase is almost never meant in this way, however. To even the most ardent supporters of such development, there is agreement that some types of uses, such as heavy industrial operations, should not be mixed with other uses, such as housing. This observation was, in fact, one of the bases for the advent of zoning, first in Germany around 1900 and later in the United States. As a result, the only uses that are considered appropriate for mixing are those that are considered to have benign influences on surrounding uses; retail and residential uses are commonly linked together, for example. Typically, as well, the focus on mixed-use development is on the mixing of uses from the different functional categories, rather than on the mixing of different types of development that exist within each category itself. For instance, the phrase generally doesn't refer to the mixing of apartments with single-family housing. Zoning codes have long prohibited multifamily housing in single-family districts, despite the benefits that such mixing might have in terms of equity (i.e., allowing people who cannot afford to purchase a house the chance to live in a larger number of areas, thereby bringing them closer to employment and services). Again, older neighborhoods that were built before zoning codes made such practices illegal sometimes have a mixture of housing types, with small apartment buildings interspersed among single-family houses. Contrary to popular belief, many such neighborhoods retain their attractiveness to homeowners, often being among the more desirable places to live (and to purchase a house) in a region.[2]

The mixing of uses can be measured at different spatial levels, including the site, neighborhood, census tract, or employment center levels (Apogee 1998). As with density, this reflects the multiple scales at which mixed use is conceptualized. At the smallest level, uses can be mixed vertically within a single building. As formerly noted, the classic formulation is the apartment unit over a small retail shop, a type of structure that used to be common in the United States (photo 8-2) and is still commonplace across Europe. Here, residents have the smallest possible distance to travel in order to access some shopping destinations: all they have to do is descend a couple flights of stairs to arrive at a bakery, corner grocery store, or restaurant. At the next spatial level larger than the individual building is the mixing of uses within a large parcel such as a suburban office development. In the typical case, services such as banks and hair salons as well as retail destinations such as lunch counters are contained within a development in order to service a large pool of office workers. Robert Cervero, a professor at the University of California at Berkeley, observes that large office developments containing no retail and service destinations contribute greatly to local traffic congestion during working hours. In such single-use developments, people have no choice but to drive during their working day in order to shop, eat lunch, and run errands. This problem is acute for suburban office centers, where the nature of the surrounding development means that distances between offices and other destinations are large, requiring long driving trips. Multiple-use office developments, Cervero notes in contrast, allow employees to make at least a portion of their midday trips on foot. They can also, theoretically, decrease the amount of land on the site that is dedicated to parking, by creating shared parking arrangements. By mixing offices with services and restaurants, the same parking lots can be used for more hours during the day, thereby decreasing the total parking allotment for the site, below what would be the sum of individual office, retail, and recreational uses (Cervero 1986, 1988).

The neighborhood or district is perhaps the most common level for analyzing the influence of mixed or separated uses. The neighborhood is the level where the mixed use concept has its most plausibility—mixing uses at this level might, so the argument goes, shift some travel that would otherwise be to destinations outside of one's neighborhood (say, from home to a shopping mall or grocery store) to those that are within neighborhood boundaries. There is, of course, much historic precedent for this line of reasoning. Many older neighborhoods, built before single-use zoning became dominant, still have the occasional small, pedestrian-oriented, and visually attractive shopping district within them. These neighborhoods are often the ones that are singled out in empirical studies as producing the greatest amount of physical

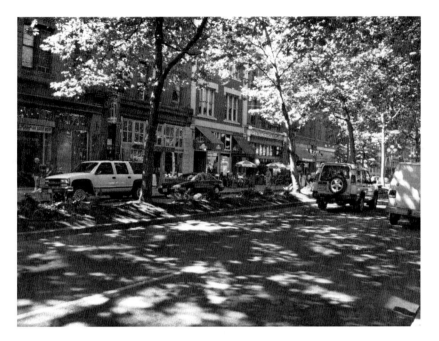

PHOTO 8-2. Vertical mixed use: apartments over retail, Pioneer Square, Seattle.

activity, in particular walking. As discussed in chapter 2, in contrast, the spread of zoning ordinances resulted in single-use development becoming the only legally allowed type of development in most parts of the United States. These neighborhoods offer little opportunity for running practical errands on foot or bicycle because there are no destinations within easy reach of housing. The exceptions are those situations in which a residential subdivision is built adjacent to a commercial district or a school; even then, obstacles may be placed between the two types of developments, breaking direct linkages between the two developments.

The mixed-use concept is also valuable at scales that are much larger than the individual neighborhood, up to and including segments of an entire metropolitan region. Jobs–housing balance, a common indicator of the degree to which uses are mixed at these scales, refers to the balance of employment and residential development across subregional boundaries (Apogee 1998). Most subregions in the United States generally suffer from a jobs/housing imbalance, where sections of the region contain the bulk of employment while others are dedicated primarily to housing (Cervero 1991). Jobs/housing balance is connected to automobile commuting, and thus the literature has tended to be dominated by research questions addressing motorized transportation. A balanced jobs/housing ratio is believed by some to reduce driving by automobile, as well as vehicle miles traveled, by shortening commute trips and reducing the degree of overlap between through and local traffic. The "bedroom community" is an example where satellite communities have developed around central cities to house workers but offer little in the way of employment. Depending upon the transportation investments that have been made, residents of such communities are often relegated to lengthy commutes. The measurement of jobs/housing balance is fraught with conceptual and methodological problems, in part because there is no widely accepted definition of the scale at which to assess the match or mismatch between jobs and housing (Apogee 1998). One problem is a limited availability of data that accurately portrays the number and type of jobs and households in subregional locations (Frank 2000). Another is the recognition that the factors that influence where people work and where they choose to live are exceedingly complex. Household structures, for example, present an unusual set of complications: in two-worker households, the decision to live in a certain place must be made with respect to not just one employment location but two.

With respect to physical activity patterns, mixed-use development has its greatest relevance at smaller scales. While regional patterns may play a larger role in influencing driving and, perhaps, mass transit usage, it is at the more localized scale where the mixing of land use patterns is likely to have its greatest influence on physical activity patterns. The linkage between transit service and walking is illustrative. While mass transit is a regional phenomenon, transit will encourage walking when the areas around the transit stations contain a sufficient mixture of uses to provide the nonmotorist with a range of destinations within a reachable distance.

Finally, a note should be made about *how* uses are mixed together. Over a given area, say an area the size of the typical neighborhood, the same uses can be mixed in very different ways. Different neighborhoods can be similar in terms of the amount of different uses that are contained within their boundaries. However, these same neighborhoods can have these different uses arranged in ways that are so different that it might influence how people travel. This phenomenon is known as "grain," defined as the "shape, size and texture of the various zones of activity" within a neighborhood, district or other spatial area (Owens 1993). The basic hypothesis is that the coarser the grain, meaning the larger the basic units within the neighborhood, the worse the neighborhood will be for physical activity. The reason is that typical large commercial and retail developments increase distances between destinations within the development itself, mostly due to the large surface parking lots that invariably accompany such development. When multiple developments with these characteristics exist within a neighborhood or district, this problem is intensified: walking distances are increased because the individual developments are set far away from other types of uses, especially residential uses. Additionally, their size also requires enormous block sizes, reducing the degree of street connectivity between destinations. Conversely, a neighborhood that consists entirely of smaller parcels will not have these problems because the smaller parcels allow for more blocks and intersections, have smaller parking lots, and shorter distances between any two buildings (figure 8-1).

Empirical Evidence

Unfortunately, most of the empirical literature on the relationships between travel and land use patterns is centered on the automobile or transit. This reflects a longstanding interest within transportation planning circles in motorized forms of transportation. There are fewer studies on the relationships between land use patterns and nonmotorized transportation. Part of the reason is the disconnect between the short nature of nonmotorized trips and the large spatial scales at which density and land use mix are typically measured. The most frequent type of study involves statistical analyses of regional or comparative travel data. For example, one study of twenty-eight neighborhoods in four California cities (Holtzclaw 1994) evaluated the effect of neighborhood characteristics, including density and land use mix, on total annual vehicle miles of travel per household. Density was found to be the most important explanatory variable of the four neighborhood characteristics examined—a doubling of residential density levels produced 25–30 percent fewer miles driven per household.

Density's influence on walking and bicycling may be felt most at higher levels of density, where the concentration of people and destinations is such that the built environment becomes the most conducive to alternative forms of travel. This hypothesis—that there is a threshold effect for nonmotorized travel—is supported by some research. For example, a study of national travel and land use data (Dunphy and Fisher 1994) found that increasing densities from a low starting point (a typical density for suburban areas) to a higher but still low level had little effect on driving and other modes of travel, including transit use and nonmotorized travel. Density's influence on behavior was modest at all levels except at the highest levels measured in the study, where the number of vehicle trips and miles driven began to fall rapidly. In contrast, at these levels the number of trips and miles by transit and by foot or on bicycle rose dramatically. Similarly, a cross-sectional study of travel behavior in Seattle neighborhoods (Frank and Pivo 1995) revealed that the relationship between density patterns and walking is nonlinear. Increasing employment density (the number of employees per acre) spurred transit and walking, but only after certain threshold densities were reached. For population density (the number of residents per acre), increasing amounts of walking and transit use were observed around thirteen residents per acre, with increases in walking above this threshold rising far more rapidly than increases in transit use. The significance of such studies is to show that density's influence on behavior may not be uniform across all levels of density; its influence may begin to be felt only when a certain critical mass of people and of destinations is reached. At this point, synergistic effects may begin to occur, wherein transit becomes more viable, walking and bicycling are feasible, and driving may become much more expensive due to the cost of parking and other factors. As real estate is extremely expensive in high-density areas, parking becomes

Facing page

FIGURE 8-1. Two examples of how mixed uses can produce very different types of neighborhood grain. The top image is the Old Fourth Ward in Atlanta, an old in-town neighborhood, containing the childhood home of Martin Luther King Jr. It is finely grained and highly walkable, with residential dwellings (gray) mixed in with mostly small civic buildings and commercial establishments (black). The transportation network consists of a fine grid system with many sidewalks. The bottom image is the neighborhood around the Greenbriar Mall in suburban Atlanta, built after World War II. This neighborhood is heavily auto-oriented due to the coarseness of its grain. The mall and other large commercial structures exist amid huge parking lots, a large arterial road cuts through the center, and housing is disconnected from commercial centers. Images based on concepts by Peter Owens (Owens 1993).

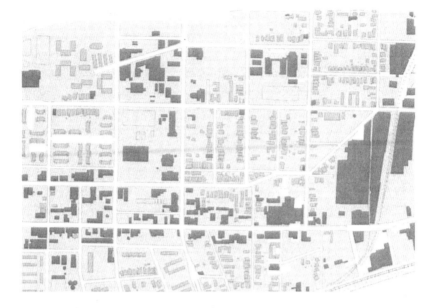

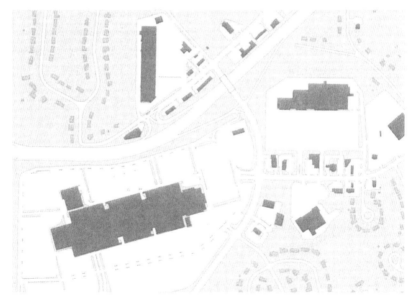

FIGURE 8-1

much more expensive, contributing to a large increase in the cost of owning and operating a vehicle—this is true in Manhattan, where only a fraction of residents own a car.

The influence of land use mix is also the subject of a good deal of study. Generally speaking, land use mix at large spatial scales has been found to have an influence on travel behavior in many studies in much the same way as density, although, admittedly, the concept is even harder to measure than density and is thus more difficult to model (Cervero and Radisch 1995; Ewing, Halidur, and Page 1994; Friedman, Gordon, and Peers 1994; Handy 1992). Mix has also been investigated at smaller scales, discussed above in the context of Robert Cervero's work. Cervero used travel patterns for employees at fifty-seven large suburban office complexes around the country to assess the impact of mixed-use development at these centers on travel behavior, finding that a greater mixture of uses increased ridesharing and reduced commuting to work via single-occupant vehicle (the mix of uses made it unnecessary to have a car for travel during the workday for many employees, thus allowing them to seek ridesharing alternatives). For travel by bicycle or on foot, moreover, the analysis showed that mix was positively and significantly related to walk and bike commuting, although only a small percent of all commuters did so by these modes (Cervero 1988).

Conclusion

Each of the land use patterns discussed in this chapter influences the utility of different modes of travel through increasing proximity between destinations. On some level, this logic is irrefutable. However, as the above discussion attests, these concepts are both more complicated in meaning and less precise in measurement than they appear upon first glance. To name just one problem, both concepts tend to be measured at a spatial level that is too large to capture much travel behavior that occurs at small geographic scales, precisely the level at which nonmotorized trips occur. As most walk trips, for example, are under a kilometer in length, a study that uses the Census tract to measure density will be unable to show how densities can vary, sometimes substantially, within the boundaries of the tract. Yet the relationship between each of these variables to travel *is* intuitively appealing and, thus, these concepts will continue to be used in transportation research. They remain irresistible because they provide a rough calculus of a place's compactness. The pattern of very low-density and single-use development in the United States hinders physical activity because it renders nonmotorized modes almost useless. It was not always so in this country. Public policies, especially zoning codes, have made obsolete the kinds of relatively high-density and mixed-use neighborhoods that used to be common in the United States and that remain common in other parts of the world. Regardless of any future successes with respect to densification and the mixing of uses, however, it must be emphasized again that land use patterns are only one part of the urban form equation in creating environments that encourage physical activity. Increasing proximity without changing both of the other two components is not likely to have more than a marginal effect on physical activity patterns.

CHAPTER NINE

Urban Design Characteristics

Every day the anxiety and depression of modern life sprang up afresh: the city is swelling, the city is filling up. The city simply builds itself anew on top of itself: the old houses towered in a cliff at the edge of the streets; the new houses still tower in new cliffs along the same streets. All the houses are on streets, the street is the basic organ of the city. . . . The whole scene is like a glimpse of purgatory.

LE CORBUSIER,
The Radiant City (1933)

What nobler agent has culture or civilization than the great open road made beautiful and safe for continually flowing traffic, a harmonious part of a great whole life?

FRANK LLOYD WRIGHT,
The Living City (1958)

Urban design characteristics represent the third major category of the built environment. These characteristics influence an individual's perceptions about the desirability of walking, bicycling, or engaging in recreational exercise at, on, or within a particular place. Most, if not all, features of the built environment constitute design elements. Unlike the motorist, a person who is walking, jogging, or bicycling is unsheltered from the elements, both human and natural. Furthermore, the distances that are typically covered while engaging in such activities are very short, at most a few miles or, frequently, only a few hundred yards. As a result, the individual is powerfully influenced by the design characteristics of their immediate surroundings—

the streets, parks, squares, plazas, buildings, lawns, sidewalks, bus stop shelters, crosswalks, trash bins, curbs, fences, billboards, plantings, and the host of other elements that together define the world we inhabit.

Yet design for the purpose of encouraging physical activity was not something that was given much emphasis during the last decades of the twentieth century. Perhaps this reflects a long-standing bias against aesthetic considerations within the discipline of city planning, a position that has roots as far back as the reaction against the City Beautiful movement at the turn of the twentieth century. Many in the then-emerging field of city planning dismissed the emphasis on aesthetics that was an inherent part of the City Beautiful movement, calling instead for a discipline based on modern, rational principles and devoted to functional considerations such as the protection of public health, the free-flowing movement of people and goods throughout the city, and the efficiency of business operations. Some have called this change a shift from the City Beautiful to what is termed the "City Efficient." What transpired, in other words, was a shift in emphasis from urban *form* to urban *function*.

Similarly, too, changes were occurring in other fields that contributed to the idea that functional rather than aesthetic considerations ought to be given more prominence with respect to urban form. As the above quotes from two of the century's greatest architects suggest, during the course of the century, especially the middle part of the century, modern architectural thought about how to design important elements of the built environment underwent something of a major change, hastened by the automobile's increasing presence. A number of architects discarded principles that had ordered basic relationships between different design elements for millennia, as technological innovations such as the automobile demanded that cities be reorganized. Many of these ideas were, as it turned out, compatible with the goals established by the new subfield of transportation engineering. At mid-century, engineers were also wrestling with the problems and opportunities created by the automobile. The singular focus on the automobile that developed within transportation engineering resulted in a consensus about design that, among other things, downgraded streets from multifaceted instruments of urban design to cogs in a functional machine with a single purpose, to move automobile traffic as efficiently as possible.

By the final third of the century, such ideas had come to dominate the design and construction of basic elements of the built environment. Only in the very last decade of the twentieth century did challenges to these ideas begin to receive widespread attention. This chapter concentrates on how the design of two basic elements of the built environment—the street and the site—has evolved over time and how each contributes to physical activity. While modern approaches to design led to streets and sites that catered to the needs and interests of motorists, during the 1990s and into the new century there was a perceptible shift toward a more comprehensive view of the design of such spaces.

Street Design

Of the two basic elements upon which this chapter focuses, streets are perhaps the most important, for they are the places where much of the physical activity in the built environment occurs. Streets are the places where people walk, jog, and bicycle most often. They form the main component of the built environment connecting destinations to one another, including destinations such as parks that might themselves be locations for physical activity. Finally, they are places where social activities can and do occur, which contribute to the basic desirability of a place for certain forms of physical activity.

The term *street design* refers to the layout and design of individual streets and street segments. The influence of street design is independent of the basic structure of the street network, that is, whether the street network is highly connected or not. A street's design can discourage walking or bicycling, for example, even though it forms a part of a fine grid network (Antupit, Gray, and Woods 1996). Streets are important design elements and have a tremendous influence on the basic fabric of any place, whether urban or suburban. As Jane Jacobs once put it, "streets and their sidewalks, the main public places of a city, are its most vital organs. If a city's streets look interesting, the city looks interesting; if they look dull, the city looks dull" (Jacobs 1993, 37). Street design influences physical activity by shaping one's desires to engage in such activity within the built environment. Here, desirability can be defined in two ways: in terms of how the street's basic design influences one's perception of safety and in terms of how it influences one's perception of the physical and social attractiveness of the street and areas immediately adjacent to the street.

Different design treatments can produce radically different settings for a person who wishes to engage in physical activity on or along the street. The street can be either dangerous and unpleasant, meaning that a person would be less likely to want to walk, jog, or bicycle along it, or safe and pleasant, which would encourage such activity.

The basic design elements of the street are represented in figure 9-1. As is shown in this figure, the definition of a "street" includes more than just the street surface itself. Not only does it include the carriageway (lanes dedicated to moving traffic) and special-purpose lanes on the street surface (for parking and/or bicycling), the definition also includes medians, tree planting strips immediately adjacent to the street surface, the sidewalk and objects on the sidewalk, and all spaces up to the private property lot line. The inclusiveness of this definition is fairly standard; urban designers tend to include these basic elements, or variations thereof, when defining the street. The mix of elements—the presence or absence of sidewalks, the number and width of street lanes, the presence of shade trees along the street—depends on the street's purpose. Among many, if not most, American traffic engineers as well as many transportation planners, street purpose is defined in functional terms having to do with moving the city's automobile traffic, measured by the number of vehicles that can be moved along the street over an hour or day. The nomenclature used to define streets within this hierarchy is itself illustrative. The streets with the heaviest traffic volumes are called arterials, while those that are slightly smaller but still carry a significant amount of traffic are called feeder streets. These names show that streets are designed with traffic flow uppermost in mind. This observation is well-founded: typically, arterials and feeders have most of the street space devoted to the carriageway and very little, if any, space devoted to medians, sidewalks, and other elements.

Anyone who attempts to walk, jog, or bicycle on or alongside most nonresidential streets in the United States knows full well how difficult, unpleasant, and even dangerous such an experience can be. It is apparent to even the casual observer that streets are places where cars rule, in terms of the amount of street space devoted exclusively to the car, the sheer number of cars on the street, and the speed of the average car traveling along the street. This is no accident. Rather, it is the result of a few important assumptions about the purposes for which a street is designed.

Streets can be said to have at least two core purposes: first, to move people

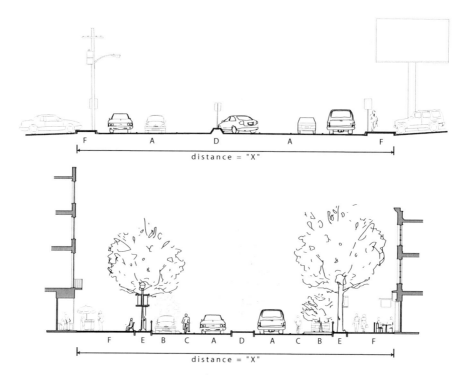

FIGURE 9-1. Street cross-sections. The upper image shows the design elements of a car-friendly street, the lower image the elements of a street designed for multiple uses. The sections are equal in width. Key: A = carriageway; B = parking lane; C = bike lane; D = median; E = tree planting strip; F = sidewalk.

and goods between destinations and, second, to serve as a stage for social interaction in a public setting (Gutman 1986). In the twentieth century, many professionals involved in urban design questions designed streets to fulfill only the first purpose. They also did so for only one type of movement, that of the motorist. Over the course of the twentieth century, responsibility for the design and construction of the nation's roads and streets became the sole province of transportation engineering, which sought to standardize the construction of streets according to seemingly objective and technical engineering principles. These principles have focused on the needs of the motorist, to the exclusion of all other users of the street and also the wider interests of the community. Among the oldest and most influential engineering societies is the American Association of State and Highway Transportation Officials

(AASHTO), whose members have had close links to road building, automotive, and trucking interest groups from its founding in 1914 forward (Ehrenhalt 1997). Since the 1950s, AASHTO has published the definitive set of design standards for the transportation engineering profession in a one-thousand-page manual titled *A Policy on Geometric Design of Highways and Streets,* but universally referred to as the "Green Book." These standards are central to understanding why most streets in the United States look and function the way that they do, for they have long been used by engineers in state or local transportation departments to design or redesign a very large percentage of the nation's roads and streets. Until 1991, federal law required Green Book standards to be used on any federally funded roadways. Basically, the Green Book's central imperative is to design streets around motorist safety and convenience, ignoring other design criteria for other users and purposes. The design standards contained in the Green Book have virtually eliminated certain types of streetscapes that enhance the experience of the nonmotorist on or along the street.

Guidelines contained in the Green Book result in two basic priorities for street design. First, the guidelines encourage the design of streets for the fast movement of traffic. Under the guidelines, engineers use the "eighty-fifth percentile" rule, wherein streets are designed or redesigned for the safety of the fifteenth fastest driver out of every one hundred on the street. In order for the fifteenth fastest motorist to be able to drive at high speeds in relative safety, inevitably the best type of street is one that is wide, straight, and level (with little elevation change). Width gives the driver enough room to safely operate the vehicle at a high speed, while straightness and a level surface provides the driver with a long and wide field of vision, necessary for safe braking distances at higher speeds (Burrington 1996). Second, the guidelines stress the importance of unimpeded traffic flow, defined in terms of the degree of traffic congestion on the street. Traffic congestion is addressed via "level of service" standards that rank stretches of roadway in terms of traffic flow performance. The level of service measure is based on a ratio, the number of vehicles distributed over a given stretch of roadway. A street segment where vehicles cannot move gets the worst grade, while the highest grade goes to a segment where cars are moving without obstruction. In many cases, streets are designed to ensure a high level of service to meet future demand, not just current demand. The level of service system is another way of formalizing street design criteria in favor of fast-moving automobile traffic. Vehicular movement trumps all other considerations, including the mobility of the auto passengers (level of service standards count the number of vehicles, not the number of passengers) as well as those outside the vehicle. Pedestrians tend to be seen as impeding the free flow of motorized traffic, for example through slowing traffic when crossing streets (Ewing 1997; Epperson 1994). American street design is, as a result, among the least pedestrian- and bicyclist-friendly in the world. In many other countries, streets are designed for slower vehicle speeds and to accommodate fewer vehicles—authorities create design guidelines that result in narrower streets, tighter curves, more sidewalks, and a much more intensive use of traffic calming devices (table 9-1).[1]

Modernist planners and architects of the early- and mid-twentieth century also shared many of the beliefs of engineers, in particular that street design parameters should be set by the needs of motorists. In their view, the street's central purpose was to move motorized traffic efficiently between the city's functional cells, between the far-flung districts (residential, industrial, and commercial) that single-use zoning had begun to impose upon the city's structure during the first decades of the twentieth century. The famed Swiss architect Le Corbusier, for example, considered the multiuse and multipurpose street to be a dangerous anachronism, out of touch with the requirements of the automobile. "Our streets no longer work," he wrote in *The Radiant City,* published in 1933. "Streets are an obsolete notion. There ought not to be such things as streets; we have to create something that will replace them." To protect pedestrians from the ravages of the automobile, he envisioned a city that not only completely separated pedestrians from vehicular traffic but also fundamentally changed the physical nature of the street in accordance with what he saw as its sole function, to move motorized traffic rapidly from place to place. In his view, the perfect city was one in which pedestrians used an extensive system of ground-level walkways while automobiles and trucks whizzed around on massive elevated roads designed exclusively for long-distance and high-speed traffic (Le Corbusier 1964).

The modern, functional view of the street as a tool for the movement of motorized traffic contradicted centuries of thought on the purposes for which a street exists. This view seriously undermined the notion that streets are legitimate public spaces for multiple uses, including nonautomotive

TABLE 9.1

Comparative street design guidelines in Britain, Australia, and the United States

Recommended design parameters/treatments	British design guidelines	Australian design guidelines	American design guidelines
Design speed	20–30 mph <20 mph (shared suface streets)	18.6–24.8 mph	20–30 mph
Pavement width	12–18 feet	16.4–21.3 feet	26 feet standard
Minimum curve radius	32.8–98.4 feet	Maximum radius specified—curves designed as traffic calming devices to limit speed	100 feet minimum—recommends larger if possible
Sidewalks	Normally on both sides; when sidewalks are not required, "shared surface" streets are built, designed to ensure a maximum speed of about 20 mph	At least one side of access (local) streets; when sidewalks are not required, authorities design streets similar to the British case	At least one side
Traffic calming devices	Raised juntions Chicanes Speed tables Street narrowings Gateways Refuge islands Bends	Chicanes Bends Refuge islands Street narrowings Humps Thresholds Roundabouts	

*Representative manuals are Residential Roads and Footpaths—Layout Considerations, Design Bulletin 32 (Britain); Australian Model Code for Residential Development; A Policy on Geometric Design of Highways and Streets (AASHTO, United States).

SOURCE: Reid Ewing, "Residential street design: Do the British and Australians know something Americans do not?" Reproduced with permission of the Transportation Research Board. In *Transportation Research Record 1455*, Transportation Research Board, National Research Council, Washington, D.C., 1994, pp. 42–49.

forms of movement along the street surface, which includes both utilitarian and recreational physical activity (walking, bicycling, jogging, rollerblading). This view, as referenced above, also completely discounted (or, perhaps more accurately, entirely ignored) the idea that the streetscape is a stage upon which social activity occurs. Social activity on the street includes planned and spontaneous activities—sitting on a bench, eating or drinking at an outdoor café table, window shopping, playing, conversing with others, dining outdoors, people watching, bumping into a neighbor for a chat, and so on. Socializing, both planned and spontaneous, tends to occur in environments that are place-specific, where people identify with a particular space and where they feel comfortable being around other people in that space; the presence of other people, in fact, is one of the key ingredients in making something—a park, square, or street—a desirable place to be (Selberg 1996; Gehl 1987). Socializing is important in its own right, contributing to social cohesion and community identity. However, it is also tremendously important with respect to physical activity. Streetscapes that encourage socializing also tend to be perfect environments for walking (photo 9-1). The view of the street as a space for social interaction rejects the idea, discussed briefly in the last chapter, that lots of people occupying the same space automatically translates into the perception that the space is crowded. In contrast, this view emphasizes the importance of having lots of people on the street in order to make the space appear lively and interesting. While there may be an absolute limit beyond which most people would define a place as uncomfortably crowded and therefore undesirable, this perspective emphasizes that having a healthy number of people in a space is a desirable feature for inducing activity.[2] A focus on the efficiency of movement completely misses this point (figure 9-2).

Modernists did know that motorists have different needs with respect to street design than other users of the street. Unfortunately, they solved this design problem by reconfiguring the street for the use of motorists and to the detriment of all others. The design of streets for multiple uses and modes requires an understanding of how the different users of the street perceive, and behave upon, the streetscape, and what needs arise from these differences. At the most fundamental level, motorists, pedestrians, joggers, and bicyclists perceive street design features differently because of the divergence in speeds at which they move along the street. The rate of speed at which one

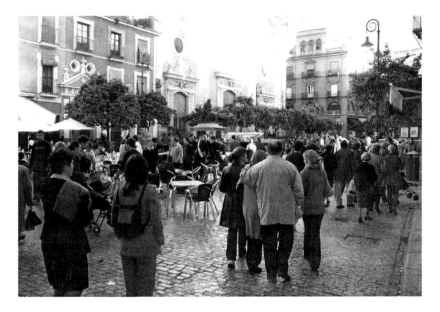

PHOTO 9-1. Highly social spaces such as the Plaza del Salvador in Seville, Spain, induce walking. People like to walk in such spaces because they are perceived as being more enjoyable, more interesting, and safer. Here, the recreational and utilitarian dimensions of physical activity are intertwined because people can perform daily tasks while also enjoying the social benefits of these environments.

is traveling will greatly determine the ability to process detail in the environment. In evolutionary terms, human senses are adapted to the speed at which humans move through space under their own power while walking. Our ability to distinguish detail in the environment is therefore ideally suited to movement at speeds of perhaps five miles per hour and under. The fastest users of the street, motorists, therefore have a much more limited ability to process details along the street—a motorist simply has little time or capacity to appreciate design subtleties. Conversely, pedestrian travel, being much slower, allows for the appreciation of environmental detail (Gehl 1987). Joggers and bicyclists fall somewhere in between these polar opposites; while they travel faster than pedestrians, their rate of speed is ordinarily much slower than that of the typical motorist.

These principles are easily translated into specific street design requirements for motorists versus nonmotorists. According to the architect Amos Rapoport, the ideal streetscape for pedestrians and bicyclists maintains the pedestrian's

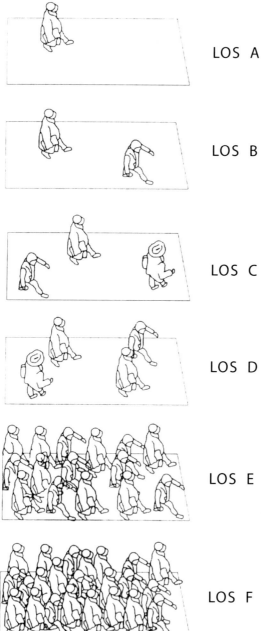

LOS A

LOS B

LOS C

LOS D

LOS E

LOS F

FIGURE 9-2. Image of pedestrian level of service standards contained in the Transportation Research Board's *Highway Capacity Manual*, a guide for transportation engineers. "Los A" is defined as the best condition; "Los F" is the worst. This figure leads one to conclude that the ideal walking environment contains a solitary individual; as shown in photo 9-1, however, the ideal pedestrian environment is highly social. Source: Reproduced with permission of the Transportation Research Board. In *Highway Capacity Manual 2000*, Transportation Research Board, National Research Council, Washington, D.C., 2000, 11–9. Original image adapted from John Fruin, *Pedestrian Planning and Design*, Metropolitan Association of Urban Designers and Environmental Planners, Inc., New York, 1971, 75, 77. Adapted from "Pedestrian Planning and Design" by John Fruin, copyright Elevator World, Inc.

visual and sensory attention at the slow speeds at which they travel. As shown in photo 9-2, designing the best street for nonmotorists requires that the street and its immediate environs contain abrupt, irregular, complex, and detailed features, with these features being interspersed at short intervals (Rapoport 1987). Streets that have bland architecture and that are dominated by long featureless horizons will not only be less interesting to the nonmotorist but will also increase the perception of the distance that one needs to cover to reach a particular destination (Gehl 1987). The street designed primarily around the speeds at which the motorist travels will be radically different. To perform tasks at high speeds safely, motorists need streets that are wide, low in visual detail, and contain no abrupt corners. The street that is ideal for nonmotorists— narrow, with abrupt changes, and a high level of detail along its edges—will not allow for safe automobile travel at higher speeds. Large, boldly stated design elements (buildings, signage, etc.) that are spaced far apart from each other and that are set far back from the street surface itself are necessary for the fast-moving motorist to be able to drive quickly and safely yet still be able to process details in the environment. The typical arterial street in the United States provides ample evidence for this hypothesis (photo 9-3). Here, all of the architectural cues of structures alongside these streets signal the influence of the street's design on everything that surrounds it. Huge billboards compete with the garish architecture of fast-food restaurants and strip malls in order to attract the motorist's attention as he or she zips past at forty miles per hour. Each design element is freestanding, with large surface parking lots separating them from each other in order to provide the necessary spacing to keep visual cues comprehensible to the motorist. It is very difficult, then, to integrate the need of motorists for fast movement with the needs of pedestrians and, to a somewhat lesser extent, of bicyclists. Only a few types of street designs can accomplish such a trick. Perhaps the most famous examples are Parisian boulevards such as the Champs-Elysées, where heavy traffic coexists alongside intense pedestrian activity. This is possible because of the enormous sidewalks on both sides of the street, the double rows of street trees, the extent and quality of street furniture on the sidewalks, and the highly detailed building facades containing pedestrian attractions (shops, cafes, etc.) that abut the sidewalk.

The design of the street surface itself—its width, the number of lanes for traffic, any provisions for on-street parking, the type of paving materials used, and so forth—is critical in determining the speed and volume of auto-

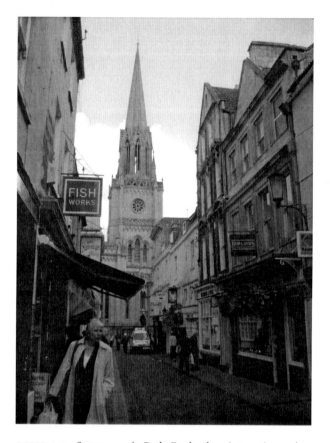

PHOTO 9-2. Streetscape in Bath, England, an interesting and
safe environment for pedestrians and bicyclists—the street is
narrow, the buildings are close to the street and have highly
detailed facades, distances between destinations are short,
signage is scaled to the pedestrian, and the horizon is enclosed.

mobile traffic upon the street. This influences the nonmotorist's perceptions
of the risk of danger from automobiles. For bicyclists, who must often share
the carriageway with automobiles, these considerations are paramount.
High-volume, fast-moving traffic represents perhaps the worst scenario for
the bicyclist, especially as streets with this type of traffic tend to carry regular truck and bus traffic as well. These conditions also have negative consequences for spaces immediately adjacent to the street, as people who are not
in vehicles tend to react negatively to the noise and stress that accompany

high-traffic and high-speed streets (Appleyard 1981; Appleyard and Lintell 1982). To enhance the nonmotorist's sense of safety, the design of the carriageway and other elements must serve to slow traffic speeds and reduce volumes, for example by reducing the carriageway width and having shorter turning radii at intersections.

The design elements that parallel the carriageway surface also have an influence on the perception of the nonmotorist. Safety can be enhanced through the ways that nonmotorized facilities are designed. Some facilities, such as wide sidewalks and bike lanes, act as physical buffers to moving traffic on the carriageway. Others make crossing the street on foot safer, such as pedestrian-friendly medians and traffic signals and well-marked, raised crosswalks (Untermann 1987).[3] Design treatments such as appropriate street lighting can also enhance safety at nighttime by making pedestrians feel safer from crime (Painter 1996). Finally, amenities such as "street furniture" add

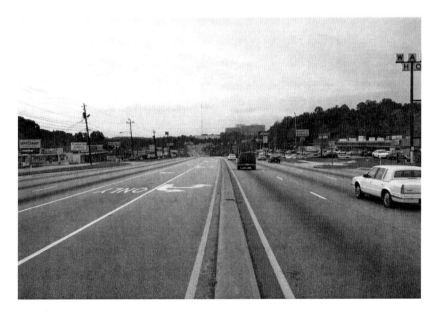

PHOTO 9-3. Streetscape in Atlanta, Georgia, the perfect environment for high-speed movement by car. The street is wide and straight, buildings are set well back from the street, architectural detail is low, distances between destinations are long, the horizon is distant, and there is no on-street parking or other hindrances (e.g., uneven carriageway surface) to impede rapid movement. The enormous scale of the signage along the street is also geared toward the motorist.

aesthetic value to the streetscape, an important consideration for someone who is not in a vehicle. Street furniture consists of interesting design touches that enhance the experience of the pedestrian, such as postal boxes, telephone booths, benches, street trees, bus stops, public art, and attractively designed street lamps (Project for Public Spaces 1993).

Fortunately, the long-standing dominance of the automobile in American street design may be eroding. There is growing pressure for acceptance of the basic premise that streets should serve a number of purposes, only one of which is the movement of vehicles. Some of this stems, of course, from complaints by pedestrian and bicycling advocates concerning road and street design. Some comes from ordinary citizens who have concerns about proposals to widen specific local roads and streets. Some comes from architects and urban designers who have reacted to modernist street design, recognizing that streets, when designed improperly, can destroy the urban fabric. Some, however, also comes from quarters where one would least expect such pressure, from a few engineering professionals as well as a small number of state and local departments of transportation. With respect to the latter groups, in 1999 the Institute of Transportation Engineers (ITE), a professional engineering society that is something of a competitor to AASHTO, released a publication containing street design guidelines for use in neo-traditional neighborhoods.[3] Design should be "specific for the particular street at hand," the document stated, meaning design for a broad set of purposes and for a streetscape defined by its architectural context. The ITE guidelines encouraged design with bicyclists and pedestrians uppermost in mind, including the provision of a full range of safety, mobility, and aesthetic design treatments for people engaging in these activities. The guidelines suggested replacing the current nomenclature for describing the street network that is used by nearly all transportation-planning agencies—arterials, collectors, and local streets. In their place, ITE proposed the use of terms such as boulevard, avenue, street, drive, and alley. The intent behind the reintroduction of these classic terms was to further the idea that streets contribute to the built environment through their design and are not just pipelines through which traffic is run (ITE 1999). Advocacy, citizen, and professional groups form a loose and diverse coalition that has organized around basic conceptual changes to street design standards. Unlike the premises behind the Green Book, "context sensitive design"—the general term given to this change in thinking regarding street design—does not elevate motorists' mobility to the highest goal. Rather, it seeks to supplement this goal with broader considerations, including design for multimodal transportation and for integrating the street into the built environment of which it is a part. In so doing, it explicitly acknowledges that engineers cannot continue to be the sole arbiters of street design. Rather, it proposes that a host of professional and nonprofessional stakeholders, including architects, environmentalists, historians, landscape architects, and citizens' groups need to be incorporated into the design process from the outset (Stamatiadis 2001; Antupit, Gray, and Woods 1996).

In 1991, after the passage of ISTEA, states were allowed to set their own design guidelines for roads built with federal funds. A few states, such as Vermont, passed design standards of their own. Some also sought to protect transportation engineers from lawsuits filed by accident victims where the accident occurred on street segments that weren't designed according to AASHTO guidelines. Vermont's law, implemented in 1997, gave engineers permission to deviate from the Green Book, including the right to design streets for lower speeds (Ehrenhalt 1997). A number of cities around the country have also begun to create guidelines oriented around design context and multimodality. In 1997, for example, Portland METRO, the metropolitan planning organization for the Portland region, issued street design guidelines consistent with these goals. Among other things, the guidelines stated that streets should accommodate multiple modes, ensure pedestrian and bicyclist safety, enhance sociability, contribute to a high quality built environment, and add to the identity of the neighborhoods in which streets are located. Further, as with the ITE guidelines, METRO outlined an alternative nomenclature for describing the street system, suggesting the use of terms such as throughway and boulevard to reflect the context-specific nature of streets (Metro Regional Services 1997). While METRO emphasized that these guidelines were not design standards, they nonetheless contributed to an erosion of confidence in the basic premises behind the Green Book standards.

There are other challenges to the dominance of autocentric street design that do not necessarily involve the rewriting of design standards. Traffic calming, for example, is an increasingly widespread practice in the United States. Traffic calming originated in Europe and it is there that it has been employed the most intensively. Starting in the late 1960s, Dutch towns began experimenting with the *woonerf* or "living yard," where neighborhood streets were transformed, through design interventions, into spaces wherein nonmotorists ruled the street and motorists had to move slowly and cautiously in order to avoid pedestrians and cyclists, rather than the other way around. Commonly, a *woonerf* scheme placed obstacles such as benches, play objects, and plantings on the street surface itself in order to require vehicles to weave in and out, at slow speeds, to negotiate the street (figure 9-3). Cobblestones and brick surfacing techniques were used to roughen the ride for vehicles. Roads were bent or narrowed, access points for vehicles were identified and their widths constricted, and strict rules for motorists were created. While *woonerven* proved to be enormously successful at slowing traffic, they were also very expensive. Nonetheless, they opened the way for a host of street design interventions between the 1970s and 1990s across northern Europe, inspiring public agencies to experiment with different types of traffic calming schemes. During the 1980s, for example, German state governments created, among other things, "Tempo 30" programs, wherein the goal was to reduce average vehicle speeds on neighborhood roads to thirty kilometers per hour (eighteen miles per hour). Measures taken included narrowing streets at critical points, creating pedestrian islands and crossings, introducing speed humps and on-street plantings, and, as in the Netherlands, introducing far stricter traffic rules (Clarke and Dornfeld 1994). Additionally, the Germans were among the first to recognize that traffic calming measures needed to be implemented across a larger area than just a single street, as such interventions tended to divert traffic to other local streets. As a result, German municipalities began creating Tempo 30 zones comprising an entire neighborhood or even larger area (Ewing 1999). Studies of areas where the Tempo 30 program was introduced have generally shown a successful reduction in average vehicle speeds as well as a decrease in accidents involving pedestrians and bicyclists.

In the United States, traffic calming was implemented later than in Europe and only within certain cities that were willing to implement it. Estimates of the number of communities that have implemented traffic calming schemes vary widely depending on the scope of the survey and the definition of "traffic calming," but it is generally accepted that a few hundred communities nationwide may have active traffic calming programs. In those areas in the United States where traffic calming has been tried, it has been implemented less intensively than in Europe, meaning that the multiple, overlapping design

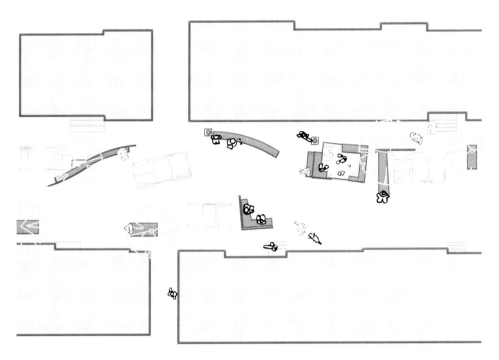

FIGURE 9-3. Overhead drawing of the design elements in a *woonerf*. Benches, sand-boxes, trees, and other obstacles are placed in the roadway to force traffic to slow to speeds that are safe for nonmotorists.

treatments found there are generally absent in the American context. Rather, frequently only one or two devices may be employed (see photos 9-4 and 9-5), often over a single street segment rather than over an entire area such as a neighborhood (Ewing 1999). To a significant degree, this is a function of the fact that Americans began traffic calming later than elsewhere. Studies from various American cities where traffic calming has been tried, most intensively perhaps in cities like Portland, Oregon, and Seattle, generally support the notion that traffic calming slows traffic speeds and reduces the number of accidents, although evidence for the latter is not as convincing. The bulk of studies from Europe, North America, and Japan show that traffic calming techniques can be very successful in achieving these goals (for a review of results, see appendix 1). Like the disconnected network, traffic calming serves to discourage through traffic. Yet traffic calming offers a major advantage over the disconnected network in the fact that it leaves connections in place for nonmotorists, thereby serving to make driving more difficult and walking and bicycling less difficult in the areas in which traffic calming schemes are introduced.

Finally, the level of service concept has also been undergoing some scrutiny. Level of service measures for pedestrian and bicycle facilities were nonexistent until fairly recently. Transportation organizations, city governments, and individuals have, however, been working to develop such standards. It is generally recognized that these standards can be helpful tools in making streets more inviting to nonmotorists. Unlike motorists, nonmotorists probably do not make decisions about which route to choose based upon the flow of pedestrian or bicyclist travel. In fact, the opposite is probably true: nonmotorists may well seek out streetscapes that have characteristics that are opposite of those sought by the motorist. Relatively crowded pedestrian spaces, for example, including pedestrian malls, squares, markets, and parks, may be desirable for pedestrian and bicycle travel. Route choice for a nonmotorist is based on a myriad number of other variables, including

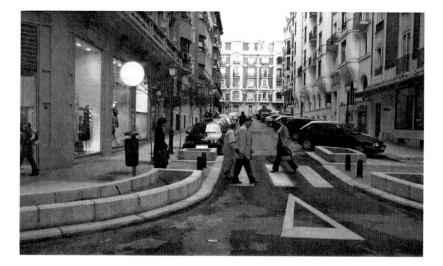

PHOTO 9-4. Multiple traffic calming techniques employed in Madrid, Spain. Here, bulbouts shorten the distance that pedestrians must travel to cross the street. The crosswalk is well marked. On-street parking is provided on both sides of the facing street, reducing the carriageway to one lane. Newly constructed planters on both street corners serve to funnel pedestrians to the crosswalk and provide a physical barrier between pedestrians and automobiles.

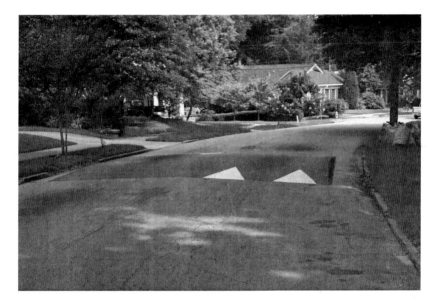

PHOTO 9-5. Traffic calming, American style. Traffic calming in the United States often consists of a single design treatment. Speed humps succeed in slowing vehicle speeds at the hump itself but otherwise fail to alter the existing streetscape.

safety, attractiveness, and distance (Highway Research Center 1994; Alexander et al. 1977). Professionals who specialize in nonmotorized transportation have been working to develop level of service measures for pedestrians and bicyclists that are based upon a more realistic understanding of how the street influences such behavior (Dixon 1995; Epperson 1994; Khisty 1994; Moe and Reavis 1997; Sarkar 1994). Aesthetic attractiveness, comfort, convenience, safety, security, and system coherence are all variables that can be included in these standards. Streets, then, are "graded" based upon performance measures for each variable: sidewalk width and continuity, the placement and design of crosswalks, the presence or absence of bike lanes, and the design of street intersections.

Site Design

Site design is important for physical activity patterns in that sites contribute to the basic attractiveness of the street as a place for physical activity. This argument rests on the principle that the streetscape is not just a linear corridor that connects destinations. Rather, the streetscape is a multidimensional space that shapes, and is shaped by, objects on its periphery. There is, in other words, a direct interaction between the street and the environment adjacent to the street (Gutman 1986). While the street is an important instrument for placing the buildings, parks, squares, and other elements of urban form along it within a particular context, these same elements also define the basic qualities of the street. Buildings, squares, lawns, parking lots, trees, and other objects that border the street give it a frame of reference. Their placement and orientation to the street influences the types of behavior among street users, motorists and nonmotorists alike.

The basic elements of the site that are important include the size of the building (width and height), the design of the building's facade, the building's orientation to and setback (distance) from the street, the placement of parking spaces on the site, and the design of the spaces between the building facade and the street. As with the design of the streetscape itself, similar principles apply with respect to the relationship between site design and physical activity. Site design elements shape perceptions of how attractive and safe the street is, which in turn influences a person's decision to walk, jog, bicycle, or socialize on the street. Sites, in other words, are important for activity along the street: streets designed with the nonmotorist in mind need to have certain types of buildings and private spaces on their edges, otherwise the fullest potential of the street as a space for physical activity will not be realized. This holds true primarily for pedestrians and for people who are interested in socializing within the confines of the streetscape, for site design most directly shapes activities that are very slow or involve no movement at all. Once again, the relationship between site design and bicycling is less straightforward. Bicyclists move at higher speeds than pedestrians and, most frequently, ride along the street surface itself (in the carriageway or special-purpose bike lanes). Bicyclists thus should be, at least theoretically, less influenced by highly detailed site designs along the street edges.

There is a widespread belief that pedestrian travel is influenced by the characteristics of buildings and other site-level design attributes (Southworth 1997; Pedestrian Federation of America 1995; Corbett and Velasquez 1994). For decades, urban designers have been pointing out the flaws inherent in buildings that are massive and featureless, designed with more regard for automobile than pedestrian access, or removed from the streetscape entirely.

It is generally asserted that in order for a building to encourage pedestrian activity, it needs to sit close to the edge of the sidewalk, have an interesting facade with design treatments that encourage interaction between the interior and exterior of the structure (such as doors, windows, stoops, porches, etc.), and not be inordinately tall or wide. Related arguments extend to the interactive effects of multiple buildings along a street; there should be small gaps (or no gaps at all) between buildings and the architectural styles should be complementary but not uniform.

From the early twentieth century on, these principles were not heeded. Planners and architects placed structures far back from the road in an attempt to ensure that fresh air and sunshine reached the interior of the structure as well as to protect the building from the dirt and pollution of the motorized traffic that ran along the street. This divorced the private sphere from the public through the introduction of a large open space between the building facade and the streetscape, one that now tends to be occupied by either large amounts of parking or by expansive lawns fronting residential and corporate property (in the words of the architect Thomas Schumacher, lawns do not "function to enclose or define street space but only to isolate the street from the house" [Schumacher 1986, 141]). A contemporaneous development was the basic design of the house itself. During the course of the twentieth century, as neighborhoods became more auto-dependent, single family houses began to be designed with porches facing the rear of the house instead of the front, as in older architectural styles (Calthorpe 1993). Front porches encouraged social and physical activity in two ways: they facilitated interaction between the residents and passersby, and their elegant designs raised the detail level of the house's facade. At the same time as designers began to place porches on the back of the house, they began to replace the front porch with the garage door—a large, featureless vertical slab on the front of the house—as the dominant design feature on the house's facade. As a result, what had been a quasi-public space (the front porch), deliberately designed to encourage social interaction, was replaced by a wholly private space (the garage) that had no relationship to the public sphere (the street).

These observations apply equally to commercial and retail site designs. Office and retail complexes have long been oriented toward the needs of the automobile user, containing linear design features, bland building exteriors, large building setbacks, significant distances between buildings, and enormous parking lots. Suburban office parks often sit behind huge lawns or are even hidden entirely from the street, buffered by large forested tracts. Retail developers site faceless, cheaply built structures behind massive surface parking lots, where the space between a development's sidewalks, if there are any, and the facade consists of an unappetizing combination of asphalt and cars. To make matters worse, these structures have few exterior features that make them interesting buildings in the first place—hence the term "big box" retail.

It should therefore come as no surprise that most contemporary retail center and office complex designs inevitably generate less pedestrian activity than older designs that were built fronting a pedestrian-oriented street. This is not just because the newer designs have uninviting spaces. They also deconcentrate destinations. The huge parking lots and general orientation of the site's buildings to one another within such complexes often create significant distances between destinations even *within* the development itself (Cervero 1986). Smaller buildings with more intricate features that are placed close together attract pedestrians because they concentrate destinations and, as a result, pedestrian activity.

Unfortunately, retail, office, and residential site design has become uniform. Regulatory and financial mechanisms impede or outright prohibit the construction of buildings that might encourage more on-street, pedestrian activity. Real estate financing, for example, is systemically biased against projects that run counter to established design formulas for shopping centers and other developments. Banks and other real estate investors evaluate projects based upon the proven track record of standard development projects. Developers will obtain financing only if they conform to established design criteria, none of which encourage pedestrian activity; for example, lending institutions often require that a shopping center's parking lot be placed in front of the building so that it can be seen easily by motorists driving past (Leinberger 2001). Moreover, developments that have pedestrian-friendly design features are more complex and costlier to build. To lenders, this translates into higher project risk and, therefore, higher lending rates (Gyourko and Rybczynski 2000). The outcome is that builders often have trouble obtaining financing of any kind for novel projects that might include, for example, a mixture of uses or a pedestrian-oriented design.

Nonetheless, in recent years many groups have called for overhauling contemporary site design practices. Peter Calthorpe laid out a number of alternative criteria for site design, all of which are designed to encourage pedestrian travel. "Buildings should address the street and sidewalk with entries, balconies, porches, architectural features, and activities which help create safe, pleasant walking environments," he wrote. "Building intensities, orientation, and massing should promote more active commercial centers, support transit, and reinforce public spaces. Variation and human-scale detail in architecture is encouraged. Parking should be placed to the rear of the buildings" (Calthorpe 1993). Many of these principles have been integrated into the New Urbanist residential developments that have actually been developed, whether done by Calthorpe's firm itself or others (Southworth 1997). Moreover, these principles have been integrated into recommendations for the wholesale redesign of commercial and retail centers, including mainstream development and real estate organizations, and have even been incorporated into some "level of service" standards for pedestrians (see, e.g., Beyard and Pawlukiewicz 2001; Jaskiewicz 1996).

Empirical Evidence

Because urban design is qualitative in nature, rigorous studies of the influence of design characteristics on behavior are rare. Much of the research into urban design, logically enough, is within the purview of architects, landscape architects, and urban designers. On-the-ground research in these fields emphasizes case studies and observational techniques. Therefore, many of the theories about design and behavior provided in this chapter are the result of insights provided from direct observation of how people react to specific surroundings.

There have been, however, a number of studies within the fields of planning and public health that have employed cross-sectional research designs that are focused on urban design variables. A public health study using Canadian data attempted to assess the relationship between environmental factors and walking to work (Craig et al. 2002). In this study, researchers created eighteen different measures of neighborhood characteristics and then rated twenty-seven different neighborhoods along each measure. Characteristics included such items as "complexity of stimulus" (amount and variety of visual and auditory stimulation, including build-ing detail and architectural variety), "visual aesthetics" (color, composi-tion, texture, and proportion of objects), and "social dynamics" (whether people could be seen moving about, sitting, and standing in the neighbor-hood). More people walked to work in the areas that had higher environ-mental scores. The relationships between social indicators (including income, education, and poverty status) and walking were not significant. A small number of other studies in the field of public health have also revealed that certain types of environments are associated with more phys-ical activity (see, e.g., Ball et al. 2001).

Within planning circles, a few studies have also been conducted that have attempted to quantify micro-scale urban design features and to assess the relationship between these variables and physical activity. A well-known study conducted in Portland, Oregon, during the early 1990s (Parsons Brinckerhoff 1993a, 1993b) offers a case in point. This study attempted to con-struct a composite variable of the pedestrian friendliness of some four hun-dred "traffic analysis zones" in and around Portland. The composite variable, termed the "Pedestrian Environment Factor" (PEF), assessed each zone using four environmental parameters: ease of street crossings, sidewalk continuity, street network characteristics, and topography. Points were assigned for each zone, with zones receiving a PEF ranking ranging from 4 (low) to 12 (high). Data from a household travel survey was then matched to the PEF rankings. The resulting data showed that zones with higher PEF's generated more tran-sit, bicycle, and walk trips, and fewer auto trips, with persons in the highest, four PEF categories making nearly four times as many walk and bike trips as households located in the bottom five categories. The study's authors also attempted to measure the effect of building setbacks on pedestrian travel in the Portland area. They gathered data for all commercial structures in three Portland-area counties in order to establish how many buildings in each of the region's traffic analysis zones were built before 1951. (The researchers believed that structures built during the decades before the 1950s were typi-cally built to the front of the lot line, rather than set back to allow for auto-mobile parking.) In areas with no buildings built before 1951, 1.9 percent of travelers walked or biked. In areas with that were over four-fifths covered by older buildings, 5.3 percent did so.

Conclusion

A primary goal of this chapter was to show that design does matter. Although, as noted, this idea is denigrated by some in the planning and engineering disciplines, the built environment has been shaped by a paradigm that is centered on designing streetscapes for the motorist convenience. Unfortunately, the street and site design guidelines and standards created and implemented over the last half century have served to create environments in which only drivers feel at home. Such regulatory and advisory devices form a large part of the explanation as to why the built environment seems to be so hostile to pedestrians and bicyclists. For example, the creation of level of service standards that are based upon vehicle-to-roadway capacity have served to downgrade alternative modes of travel, both within transportation planning and engineering circles as well in reality, on the ground. The level of service standard is an important tool driving transportation funding allocations. Because the methodology that has been erected in support of the level of service standard has emphasized the improvement of traffic flow along congested street segments, transportation dollars are prioritized for automobile travel at these locations. Until a new system for multiple modes of travel is devised, containing the same level of rigor and engendering the same amount of respect in engineering and planning circles, arguments for sufficient funding for nonmotorized investments will continue to be met with considerable resistance.

CHAPTER TEN

Application of Principles

DATA FROM SEATTLE AND ATLANTA

The foregoing chapters have established the logical and empirical relationships between the built environment and physical activity, in particular utilitarian forms of physical activity. The research that is summarized in these chapters provides evidence that walking and bicycling increase in certain types of environments and decrease in others. Yet an important part of the equation is missing, that which links the built environment to overall levels of physical activity as well as health outcomes. It is not a given that where people walk or bicycle for utilitarian purposes will also be places where overall physical activity levels are higher. Residents of auto-oriented neighborhoods may drive to parks and other neighborhoods that are more walkable and walk there. Or they may take a large number of walks for recreational purposes only within their neighborhoods and not report these activities as trips within regional travel surveys. Therefore, these activities may not get recorded and assessed in studies of travel behavior and physical activity. As a result, we can state that past research provides a linkage between the built environment and travel but leaves open the question as to connections between the built environment and physical activity. Moreover, there is little direct evidence on what types of connections exist between the built environment and health precursors such as obesity. Yet because public health problems such as obesity have become so important, clarifying these linkages is sorely needed. From a policy and decision-making perspective, it is important to know the health related outcomes of an emerging set of interventions drawn from combinations of physical changes to local and regional land use and transportation investment decisions.

Linking Health with the Built Environment

New findings are reported here that extend existing research linking the built environment to physical activity and obesity. While preliminary in nature, the findings from this research suggest that important relationships do exist between the built environment and physical activity and health. It also illuminates the complexities that exist when attempting to systematically link the built environment with activity patterns and health outcomes. In short, the science is somewhat embryonic. However, a recent review of empirical research from these two literatures, planning and health, suggests significant relationships do exist between the built environment and predictors of health (Saelens, Sallis, and Frank). More research will be required to understand how specific types of interventions impact overall levels of physical activity per person and per household, in particular to dissect these relationships for specific demographic groups as defined by income, race, age, and so on. Furthermore, additional studies will be required that address the underlying attitudinal factors that impact physical activity and the self-selection of specific populations into walkable and auto-oriented communities.

This chapter provides a summary of findings from research conducted by the authors and others within the Atlanta and Seattle regions that point to certain relationships between the built environment, levels of activity, and overweight and obese status. Research results from Seattle describe the specific types of land use patterns that are correlated with walking and biking for work and non-work purposes. These findings are supplemented by additional results from two communities in San Diego and for a cohort of nine hundred Medicaid recipients in the Seattle region. Collectively, these studies are among the first efforts to test how the physical environment that people live in relates with objective and self-reported levels of physical activity. In Atlanta, research findings are presented that links the level of obesity with the residential environments of 12,169 residents in the sprawling Atlanta region. This new data is part of the SMARTRAQ research program and is the first major effort to include the reporting of body mass index and physical activity patterns of respondents within a major regional household travel survey. SMARTRAQ provides a model for other regions to follow that links travel and activity patterns, land use and transportation systems data, and physical activity and health characteristics. It is a significant step to cross-disciplinary boundaries between city planning, transportation engineering, and public health and is backed by a partnership formed between agencies from these different arenas.

Why Do We Walk?

Results from Seattle are based on the 1999 Puget Sound Activity Survey, a regional travel survey conducted by the Puget Sound Regional Council as part of that region's ongoing transportation planning program. The resulting six-thousand-household survey database provides detailed information on the travel and activity patterns of these households. The authors conducted research to assess how the land use and transportation patterns in the areas surrounding these households affected the frequency of walking for residents. The findings indicate that the choice to walk for nonwork travel is a function of the numbers of different types of retail and commercial land uses within our own neighborhood—and less a function of the amount or floor area devoted to these nonresidential land uses. Specifically, walking for nonwork purposes is most highly correlated with the numbers of retail establishments, restaurants, and office buildings within a quarter mile of where we live (Frank, Dumbaugh, and Leary 2002). To a slightly lesser extent, the choice to walk is also associated with the numbers of schools and grocery stores.

While these findings may seem intuitive, previous research focused primarily on the amount of commercial or complementary uses, and less so on the scale at which these uses are built. How uses are mixed, it seems, are as important as the aggregate amount of mixture, a finding that reinforces the idea of neighborhood "grain" that was introduced in chapter 8. Pedestrians seem to respond differently to the different scales at which uses are mixed; for planners, this means that measures should be created that lean away from the amount of square feet of different uses and toward the absolute number of different commercial land uses within a community. This research is also significant because it prioritizes specific types of uses and their relative contribution toward the choice to walk within communities and offers planners and activists a basis for lobbying for certain types of uses within local communities. It is interesting to note that this research found that the frequency of walk-

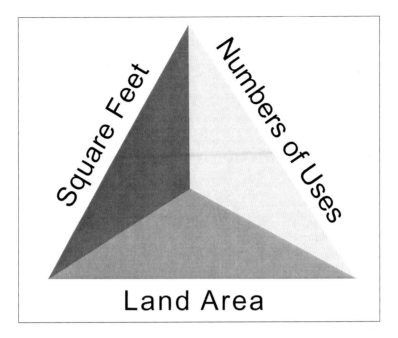

FIGURE 10-1. A land use triangle showing the multiple dimensions of land use mix that influence walking: the numbers of different types of uses, the square footage of each type of use, and the land area devoted to recreational spaces. Data from Seattle suggests walking may be more a function of having a large number of different types of uses near home and less a function of the amount of square footage dedicated to these uses. The land area devoted to recreational uses (parks) is also less significant, but this may be more the result of how nonmotorized recreational trips are collected in travel surveys.

ing was not as strongly related with the amount of land area devoted to open space and recreational use (e.g., parks) within a neighborhood. While this is a potentially significant finding, suggesting as it does that park space is not a significant predictor of one type of physical activity, it may also be an artifact of how "destination-based" transportation data is collected. Naturally enough, regional travel studies focus on trips and therefore are constructed to capture only utilitarian travel by respondents. There is a reduced emphasis upon nonpurposive forms of travel or exercise such as jogging. As a result, pedestrian trips made for a recreational or health-related benefit, like a walk around the block after dinner, are most often not captured in such studies.

These findings from Seattle are illustrated with the help of a land use triangle, shown as figure 10-1, which expresses land use in terms of three dimensions—numbers of uses, square feet, and land area across a variety of uses. Whereas the numbers of uses matter most in predicting the choice to walk for nonwork travel, land area devoted to recreational use or park and open space may be the most important predictor of the choice to walk for recreational activities. This latter hypothesis may be subject to the same dynamics as those that surround utilitarian travel patterns. Therefore, the land use triangle provides a "surface" bounded by these three fundamental dimensions of land use.

For illustrative purposes, we have provided a comparison of two households in the Seattle Region with similar incomes and ages but differing land use patterns. One is located in a finely grained and mixed use neighborhood known as Queen Anne Hill and the other is located in a single use community that was recently developed near Lake Sammamish (figure 10-2). Among other qualities, the Queen Anne Hill neighborhood offers more civic amenities and services near this household than does the more suburban Sammamish community offer its residents. While this comparison between these two households is solely for illustrative purposes, it nonetheless illuminates the divergent land development patterns and resulting travel choices that are expressed within these two settings. Both households have similar incomes and are of similar ages, yet residents of the more urban Queen Anne Hill household walk far more and drive far less than the suburban Sammamish counterpart.

The Built Environment and Physical Activity— An Emerging Agenda

The relationships between urban form and physical activity are confounded by the fact that many forms of physical activity, like working out at a gym or swimming, are structured and do not occur within the confines of the built environment, meaning that they are private activities that are conducted at home or in a health club. Moreover, most surveys designed to measure levels of physical activity have relied on self-reported information from respondents, a method that introduces considerable inter-respondent variation in reporting accuracy. To overcome these problems, social scientists have begun using accelerometers (devices worn by the respondent that capture the respondent's rate of movement using a sensor or gyroscope) to provide objec-

Queen Anne Hill   Lake Sammamish

Queen Anne Hill		Lake Sammamish
38 years	*Average Age*	37 years
$79,500	*Median Income*	$80,200
3	*# Household Members*	4

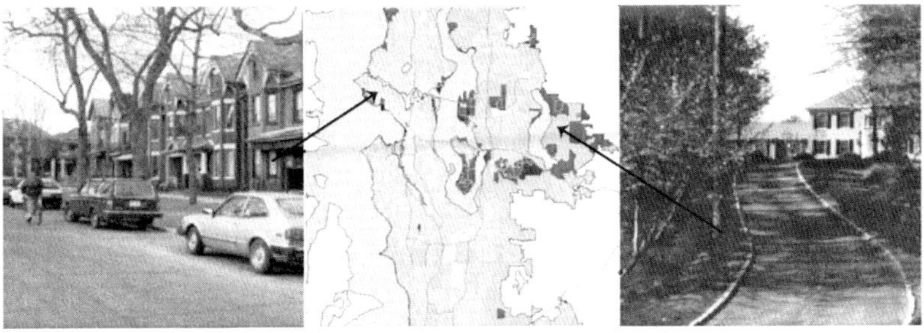

Travel Choice

	# Trips over 2 days	
26	*# Trips over 2 days*	46
31%	*Drive*	86%
8%	*Schoolbus*	14%
61%	*Walk*	0%

Neighborhood Land Use

76%	*Residential*	100%
22%	*Civic*	0%
2%	*Retail*	0%

FIGURE 10-2. Comparison of travel patterns for two families living in different parts of the Seattle region. Queen Anne Hill is an older, more urban neighborhood, while Lake Sammamish is a newer neighborhood in the suburbs. This image is illustrative only.

tive measurements of physical activity patterns. Several studies currently underway are deploying accelerometers in an attempt to use this technology to overcome these dual problems—first, to gauge when people are getting physical activity (i.e., accelerometers are useful in that they allow all kinds of physical activity to be captured, regardless of where and how the activity is done) and, second, to accurately record levels of physical activity without depending on self-reported information. The hope is that resulting data about overall activity patterns can be broken down and analyzed by type of residential environment.

For instance, a pilot study comparing activity levels between the residents of the Clairemont and Normal Heights communities in San Diego used accelerometers in order to gather such information (Saelens et al. forthcoming). The authors found that residents of the more walkable Normal Heights are indeed more physically active overall than residents of the less walkable Clairemont community. The study concluded that the higher levels of physical activity observed in Normal Heights was in the form of moderate activity associated with walking and not with vigorous activity, which appeared to be relatively constant between the residents of similar age and income within these two communities. Additional data collected within the context of a different city (Seattle) and study group (the Group Health Cooperative, using 900 households) supports these findings. Households located within the most walkable communities within the Seattle region stated that they were more physically active and walked more frequently than did those residents who lived in the region's least walkable environments (Schmid and Frank 2003).

Linkages with Obesity

While findings such as these suggest that the built environment impacts how and where we are likely to walk, and that overall levels of physical activity are higher in more walkable environments, there still remains no direct linkage with health or any precursors of health impairment such as obesity. Much has been written about the alarming increase in the levels of obesity in Americans in the last two decades of the twentieth century. Contemporaneous with increasing weight is a decline in the proportion of trips made on foot (Federal Highway Administration 1997). However, to date no study has been able to draw a direct connection between increasing overweight and obesity, declining trips made on foot, and the characteristics of the built environment.

To test these relationships, the Atlanta based SMARTRAQ program collected height and weight characteristics from the members of households that participated in a travel survey of that region. Household addresses were provided, which enabled a direct correlation to be tested between the built environment surrounding each household and body mass index (BMI).

Land use measures were estimated based on the range of destinations that could be reached within a kilometer network distance from survey households. Figure 10-3 conveys two types of buffers (network and crow fly) within two different settings in Atlanta, one urban and one suburban. Crow fly buffers are based on a direct distance from one's house and result in a perfect circle. Network buffers are irregular in shape and size and articulate that area that can be accessed within a given distance on the street network from a given point such as a survey household. The urban network buffer shown in figure 10-3 is a larger proportion of the crow fly buffer than its suburban counterpart. This is because it has a more connected street network which, in turn, increases the potential for shops and services to be within walking distance.

In our most recent research using the SMARTRAQ data, we have found significantly lower obesity rates for those who reside in more compact, denser, more pedestrian friendly and transit supportive areas of the Atlanta region. Figure 10-4 reports some of these findings for white males for this region and illustrates that the proportion of white men that are obese declines from 23 to 13 percent as density increases from the lowest (0–2) to the highest (8 and up) dwelling units per acre.[1] We chose to display white men because the rate of decline in obesity was stronger than we found in women and black men. Further investigation, which adjusted for other factors that impact obesity including age, income, and educational attainment, confirmed that higher levels of residential density are associated with a reduced likelihood of obesity for white men. Moreover, after adjusting for effects of age, income, and educational attainment, our results also found that the level of land use mix, or availability of commercial and retail uses where one lives, was found to be associated with a reduced likelihood of being obese for white males and females and for black males. In fact, at the margins, the probability for a black male to be obese declines from 0.34 to 0.11, a threefold reduction in the likelihood of obesity.

Our data further suggest that this reduction in the likelihood of obesity in higher-density and mixed-use areas is due in part to higher levels of physical activity in these areas. After adjusting for age and income, the data shows significant positive relationships between self-reported levels of physical activity for white males and females in more compact and mixed-use environments. Moreover, it also shows a very strong relationship between the amount of walking that is reported for nearly all populations in more compact and mixed use environments. As noted, the strength of the positive relationship between self-reported levels of moderate and vigorous activity and the choice to walk was far greater for white males and females. Therefore, we

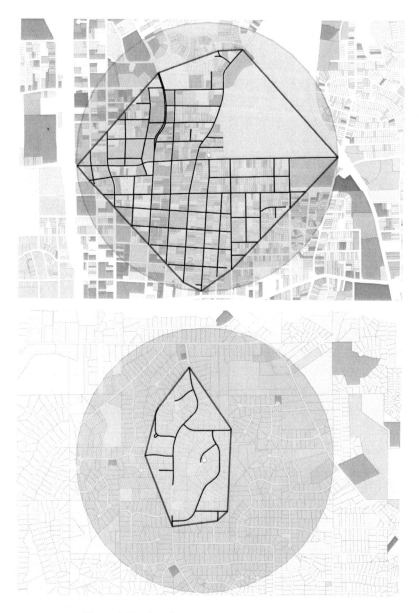

FIGURE 10-3. Two neighborhoods in Atlanta: Midtown (upper figure) and a sub-urban neighborhood (lower figure). In addition to differences in land use patterns, these neighborhoods also differ dramatically in terms of connectivity. The network buffers in both figures show the distance a person could travel *on the road network for one kilometer* from the center of the diagram, while the crow-fly buffers represent a one-kilometer straight-line distance from the center. The polygon for Midtown occupies a much larger fraction of the one-kilometer circle, indicating how much easier it is to get around this neighborhood.

suspect that at least part of the association between land use patterns and BMI in whites is explained by the impacts that these land use factors have on physical activity patterns. Data shown here support the hypothesis that supportive built environments can have direct health-related benefits in terms of an increased likelihood of being active and reduced likelihood of being obese and predisposed to known health risks associated with obesity. Yet the exact nature of the connections between these phenomena remains unclear. Of course, we acknowledge that other considerations such as attitudes; distributions of grocery stores, quality eateries, and fast food outlets; and predispositions to being physically active are at play. Additional research needs to be, and will be, conducted to explain the variations between white and black, and male and females shown in these results, some of which are cultural and others that are socioeconomic in nature.

Conclusion

Emerging research is providing ways to better understand how the built environment influences our choice to walk, our levels of physical activity, and even to some extent, our weight. While findings presented in this chapter are preliminary in nature, they collectively begin to weave some important threads between travel choice, activity patterns, and important precursors to our health. Significant research has been conducted affirming that higher levels of BMI predispose populations to several chronic ailments including type 2 diabetes and cardiovascular disease. Research presented herein begins to document the critical link between the built environment and physical activity patterns—and supports the argument that connections can be made from the built environment to health via physical activity. However, far more research will be required before any claim can be made as to the nature of such a relationship. To this end, this research is just the beginning of findings that will be forthcoming from several major efforts currently underway to gain a better insight into how our physical environment impacts our physical well-being. For example, at the time of this writing, data is being collected in several regions of the nation to more systematically relate the built environment with objective measures of physical activity. Other data collection is being done suggesting that residents of more compact and interconnected portions of the Atlanta region know their neighbors better and have a better sense of

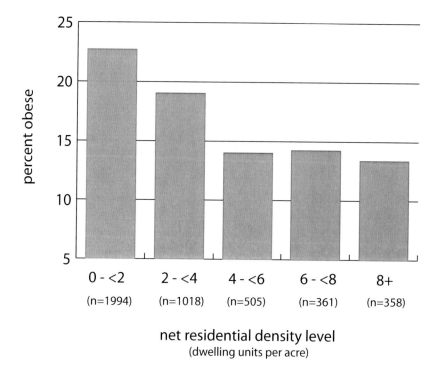

FIGURE 10-4. Percent obese for white males by net residential density levels, Atlanta, Georgia. Obesity = Body Mass Index grater than 30 kg/m^2.
SOURCE: SMARTRAQ research program data, 2002. N=4.23.

their communities than residents of more dispersed and disconnected environments. Perhaps more than anything else, it is the ability to traverse formerly impermeable disciplinary boundaries that makes it possible to begin to unravel the complexities at play between human behavior and the built environment that we have studied.

CHAPTER ELEVEN

Conclusion

In the opening chapter of this book, we observed that there is an increasing amount of criticism of the dominant types of development in the United States. It seems, moreover, as if this criticism is arising from all quarters, not only from those whom one would suspect would be at the forefront of concerns about cities, such as planners and architects. A wide array of people, including environmentalists, journalists, social justice advocates, public health officials, and ordinary citizens are expressing dissatisfaction with the built environment that we inhabit. What all of these critics share is a sense, albeit an inchoate one, that the built environment as it has been constructed is dysfunctional and that a new set of solutions is needed to correct a host of significant problems. One of the newer sources of concern, we have asserted in these pages, has to do with the problem of physical inactivity. To the extent that this book has defined this problem as a matter of public health and has illuminated some of its built environment causes, the next logical step is to address the policy mechanisms that perpetuate the dominant types of development in this country.

Many people assume, erroneously, that the built environment that we inhabit—the sprawling, horizontal, auto-dependent form that constitutes the default way of building—is the result of our market economy operating at its finest, representing, in the aggregate, individual preferences for things like single-family houses and cul-de-sacs and strip malls. While there is, undoubtedly, some truth in this assertion, there is also more than enough historical as well as contemporary evidence to point to a very different conclusion, namely, that public policies have had, and continue to have, tremendous influence in shaping these growth and development patterns. It is now an accepted part of the "smart growth" lexicon that federal, state, and local policies have greatly encouraged sprawl in this country. A recent analysis of the Urban Land Institute's national membership database found that local government development regulations were a primary barrier steering developers away from mixed-use projects and other smart growth approaches to development (Inam, Levine, and Werbel 2002).

Federal housing and transportation policies, engineering codes adopted by state departments of transportation, and municipal zoning and subdivision codes are just a few of the policy mechanisms that have fueled modern development. Policies at the federal level have provided much of the force behind modern development patterns. Many, for example, have criticized federal transportation and housing policies for feeding sprawl. It is now generally accepted that the federal housing policies that were constructed in order to get the housing industry through the Great Depression proved to be powerful enablers of the postwar suburban housing boom. The mortgage insurance program under the FHA, for example, was aimed at subsidizing the purchase of single-family homes, not at multi-family housing or rentals of any kind. Through the rating systems that the FHA created, certain types of neighborhoods—especially those containing renters and multi-family housing—were given a higher risk rating and therefore were not eligible for FHA loan guarantees (Jackson 1985).

Land use policies at other levels of government also have been major contributors to the problem. As discussed in chapter 2, the zoning movement arose in the early part of the twentieth century because planners believed that lower residential densities and a separation of uses needed to be mandated by government action. Little has changed in the intervening decades, as such regulatory devices have contributed, in a systematic fashion, to low-density development on the regional periphery (Pendall 1999). Yet modern zoning, like the early history of zoning in the United States, has its constitutional basis in health, safety, and welfare considerations, a fact that makes this tool one of the most powerful for changing land use development practices; what is required is not an elimination of zoning but, rather, a reform of the zoning codes themselves. Other state and local policies also have direct and indirect influences on land use patterns. Many states have rules requiring minimum acreages for new school construction, where new schools must provide a significant amount of floor space for each student. In practice, this has meant that school boards find they have no choice but to build new schools in outlying areas where land is cheap. Additionally, school funding formulas and building codes tend to work against the refurbishing of schools in older neighborhoods, instead serving to favor the construction of new schools. While the goals that underscore such policies often are admirable—acreage requirements, for example, are intended in part to give children enough space for play and exercise—the result is that these policies both promote exurban development (in essence, by facilitating the construction of public infrastructure in rural areas) and further decrease the odds that a child will be able to walk or bicycle to school (by eliminating older schools in walkable neighborhoods and creating a fewer number of large schools in newer residential areas).[1]

Federal and state transportation policies and funding also provided the basic infrastructure around which auto-oriented development occurred. The federal government funded the Interstate system, of course, and provided much of the money for a host of other major highways. Additionally, billions were and are spent every year by state governments on nonfederal highways and roadways. Altogether, today these systems comprise a dense network of thousands of multilane highways and roads, constituting the basic infrastructure upon which people drive to and from work, schools, and services. But the impact of these transportation dollars is not felt just in terms of the infrastructure *for* motorists, it is also felt in the relative neglect of infrastructure for other modes and the marginalization of all other means of surface transportation. During the postwar era, public funds for roads have outstripped funds for transit and intercity rail by a ratio of perhaps ten to one or even more.[2] For investment in walking and bicycling systems, this ratio reaches absurd proportions: while comprehensive statistics on this topic are difficult to come by, it is safe to claim that federal and state spending on roadways during the postwar period has far exceeded a trillion dollars, while funding for walking and bicycling projects, in contrast, might total one to two billion dollars, or less than a thousandth of the amount that has been allocated to highways. Federal funding for such projects wasn't even available until 1973, when the Federal-aid Highway Act of that year allowed states to use a small percentage of funds to construct separated systems; over the subsequent two decades, twenty states spent a total of $41 million under this program

(Lipford and Harrison 2000). During the 1990s, with the passage of two landmark transportation bills, ISTEA (1991) and TEA-21 (1998), this situation changed for the better, as bicycle and pedestrian projects became eligible for funding under a broader set of categories.[3] Yet despite a massive increase in funding for such projects as a result, the amounts are still extremely modest compared to spending on traditional types of highway construction and repair. Many states have failed to spend anything approaching the maximum amount allowable under ISTEA and TEA-21 for these projects, preferring to continue spending as much as possible on road building.[4]

The Need for Policy Integration

What is remarkable about these disparate areas of public policy is the degree to which they reinforce one another in terms of practical outcomes. This is because, as we argued in chapter 2 as well as elsewhere in this book, each type of policy has worked toward the same set of goals with respect to how the built environment ought to be arranged: during this period, policy goals have been directed at producing built environments that are low in population as well as structural densities, have their uses separated from one another, and depend upon an auto-oriented infrastructure in order to function. These seemingly disparate sets of policies, therefore, work in concert with one another.

This simple observation demonstrates that individual policies often have influence across boundaries. Figure 11-1 illustrates this basic point. In the figure, three spheres overlap—transportation investments, policies, and patterns (meaning highway funding, engineering standards, etc.); land development policies and patterns (meaning zoning codes, subdivision regulations, housing policies, policies for the acquisition of greenspace for parks, etc.); and public health policies and outcomes (meaning the array of policies within federal and state health agencies). While each sphere is independent of the others in some ways, they all are related in others. In the figure, the lightly shaded areas illustrate binary relationships. For example, land development policies and patterns have relevance to transportation policies and patterns because, as was discussed in chapters 7 and 9, different types of development shape different travel patterns among individuals. When developers conform to subdivision regulations that require low connectivity

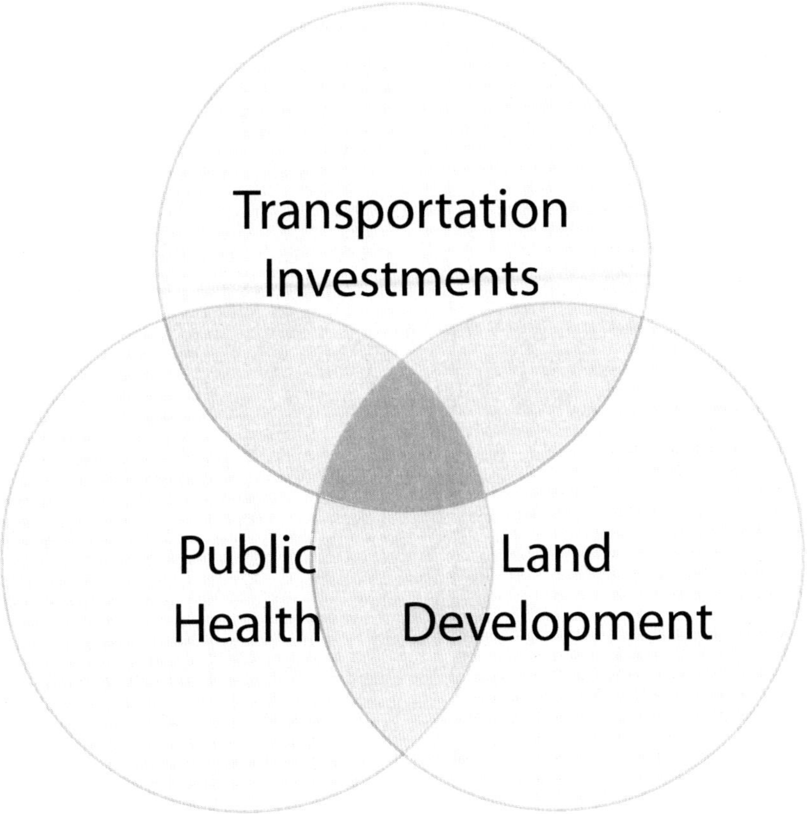

Transportation
Investments

Public   Land
Health   Development

FIGURE 11-1. Interaction across policy spheres

and to zoning codes requiring large lots (hence low population density), they are contributing to regional transportation problems by forcing more drivers onto the same number of arterials. Simultaneously, federal and state transportation policies and funding are geared toward providing an extensive road infrastructure, thereby enabling developers to access undeveloped rural areas for the purposes of building new developments. Similarly, both health-related behaviors and health outcomes are related to policies and developments in each of the other spheres.

The key challenge is to harmonize policy agendas across all three spheres. Without such harmonization, any curative proposals may address only one or two dimensions of the problem. For instance, many developments that are labeled as New Urban represent, from the standpoint of public health, movement in a positive direction; built with the nonmotorist in mind, such developments are one attempt to address the ill effects of contemporary subdivision design. New Urban design philosophy stresses the importance of mixing uses, building pedestrian-friendly streetscapes, and adding other design touches such as village squares in order to give people a reason to walk or bicycle within the confines of the development as well as giving them a sense of attachment to their community. However, to the extent that many of these developments tend to be located on the suburban and even exurban fringe of a region, nearly the same set of objections can be leveled against this model of development as against standard subdivision design. While such development on the regional periphery may allow some local, nonwork trips to be done on foot or by bicycle, the basic transportation equation remains unchanged—longer journeys, including the commute to work but also including many cross-regional shopping trips and other errands, remain completely dependent upon the automobile. These projects offer only a partial solution, as the relative merits and demerits of transit and nonmotorized modes versus automobile travel remain unchanged for longer trips.[5] Such design solutions, focused as they are on the immediate environs of the upper-income residents of these developments, continue to add to a host of regional problems, including but not limited to poor air quality and inequitable development patterns.

To solve the public health problems to which the built environment is a significant contributor, policies will have to be shaped so as to address both the "how development is designed" and the "where development goes" questions that are at the center of the problem. The design template regarding how private development ought to proceed is not, we believe, terribly complex: at the neighborhood level, it should be oriented more around the needs of the pedestrian and the bicyclist and less around that of the motorist. To some extent, this position echoes the thesis advanced by Clarence Perry in the 1920s, where the neighborhood's internal organization was designed with the pedestrian, especially the child pedestrian, at its center. Yet, even if such neighborhoods wholly replaced the existing subdivision template in the United States, if development were to continue apace on greenfields at the exurban fringe of a region, progress would be made but it would not be a complete solution. Such development would perpetuate the reliance on the automobile and do little for air quality, not to mention automobile congestion on major highways and arterials.

This is the "where" problem of development and speaks to the need to create policy instruments that make infill development and, critically, infill *re*development so important. To simultaneously get people to be more physically active, clean the air, and reduce congestion, the synergistic relationships between land use patterns, transit, and nonmotorized forms of travel need to be recognized (or, more accurately, reaffirmed) and enhanced through intelligent public policies. Whereas nonmotorized modes of travel are highly localized in nature (given the inherent distance limitations involved in travel on foot or by bicycle), transit provides regional accessibility for the nonmotorist; when done properly, as is the case in many cities in the Netherlands, Germany, Switzerland, Japan, and elsewhere, transit service can greatly enhance the feasibility of nonmotorized modes.

What is needed is an agenda for research and policy change that recognizes the interactions between these spheres. For instance, there is an ongoing and vigorous debate concerning the relationships between transportation patterns, land development patterns, air quality, and adverse public health outcomes (in the form of respiratory problems and diseases). While, of course, it has long been known that poor air quality has adverse impacts on public health (this is the major reason why there is a Clean Air Act), it was only during the 1990s that the relationships between all of these factors, transportation and land use patterns included, began to be assessed in earnest. Automobile and truck emissions are increasingly large contributors to poor air quality—in many regions of the country pollution from motor vehicles exceeds that from point sources (factories and power plants)—and many have been modeling the connections between these sets of variables (see, e.g., Freedman et al. 2001; Frank, Stone, and Bachman 2000; Tolbert et al. 2000).[6] More importantly perhaps, such research has had an influence on—as well as being influenced by—actual policy changes. For example, Congress broadened the scope of transportation policy (through ISTEA, passed in 1991) to require states and regional planning agencies to demonstrate that transportation investments would not result in violations of the Clean Air Act. Moreover, under the Clean Air Act Amendments passed in 1991, Congress mandated that states and regional planning agencies show that their transportation plans and investments conformed with a preestablished emissions budget for automobiles and trucks. By the end of the decade, the Environmental Protection Agency had begun to explore how states and planning agencies could get credit, to be applied against their emissions budget, for adopting innovative land use practices.[7] Research is needed to clarify how strategies promoting nonmotorized transport and reducing regional air pollution levels can be extended to mitigate greenhouse gas formation. Housing policy, too, has shown signs of movement toward a model that emphasizes the areas of coincidence between housing and transportation patterns. During the late 1990s, a group of nonprofit organizations began advocating a new policy instrument called Location Efficient Mortgages (LEMs), the intent of which is to reward homebuyers who choose to buy in dense urban areas near transit. The idea was that because purchasing a home in this type of neighborhood would save on transportation expenses (i.e., less money would be spent on automobile-related costs), the consumer ought to be able to afford a larger mortgage. FannieMae, the nation's largest home financing organization, has created a LEM pilot program.

Additionally, there are a slew of small but meaningful changes that can make existing places more conducive to physical activity. Even tiny funding reallocations within transportation agencies, for example, could make a big difference with respect to the opportunities for physical activity within existing development. Relatively minor amounts of money dedicated to building high-quality amenities for pedestrians and bicyclists at key locations, for example at major intersections, would remove a considerable amount of risk for traveling on foot or by bicycle. Footpaths and bicycle paths that are placed between proximate-but-disconnected developments would link more destinations for people interested in taking these modes. There are many such examples, including pathways within subdivisions (linking cul-de-sacs one to another, for example) and pathways between residential subdivisions and malls or other commercial spaces.

While all of these changes in public policy are helpful, taken together they amount to only a fraction of the changes that are needed if the built environment is to be made more conducive to physical activity at a whole-sale level. Unlike respiratory diseases, which have been linked in federal and state policies to environmental conditions for several decades, physical activity tends to be viewed by policy makers and laymen alike through an individualistic prism, not an environmental one. Part of the reason is that over most of the last half century there was no urgent need to link the built environment to physical activity patterns. For years, public health research focused on vigorous physical activity instead of moderate activity, which meant that the forms of moderate activity that have been the subject of most of the discussion in these pages—walking and bicycling—were not emphasized. Additionally, until the 1980s public health agencies generally did not focus on the spatial context in which many health problems arose. When coupled with a lack of emphasis on walking and bicycling within transportation planning and other fields, it was perhaps inevitable that the question of how the built environment influences physical activity patterns would be a marginal one.

Admittedly, it will be difficult to construct a policy edifice that encourages the creation of physical-activity-friendly environments. Mechanisms will need to be found to change land use practices at the local level so as to make the built environment more hospitable for pedestrians and bicyclists—zoning codes need to be changed to allow higher densities and a mix of uses, subdivision regulations will need to mandate shorter setbacks, narrower streets, and so on. State and local governments will have to plan for, and find the funds for, more public recreational facilities, such as parks, ball fields and open space. Transportation agencies will need to be cognizant of the impact that their policies and funding levels have on discouraging walking and bicycling (perhaps, for instance, by incorporating a "health impact statement" into their procedures for assessing the merits of transportation investments, similar to the environmental impact statements that are currently required under federal law), while an array of other policies at the federal and state level will need to be reexamined for their effects on physical activity.

The shifts that are being suggested here will require a transformation in thinking across many policy areas and within all levels of government. Other countries have invested heavily in an alternative development paradigm, constructing fewer roads and more transit, allowing and even mandating higher densities and a mixture of uses, purchasing large amounts of greenspace for parks and urban forests, and, perhaps most importantly, taking walking and bicycling seriously enough to warrant significant investment in infrastructure for these types of travel. Even within our own history, important changes in thinking about how to design and build cities have occurred on a number of occasions. Zoning, for example, didn't exist on a widespread basis in the United States until the 1920s and 1930s, when most municipalities adopted codes over a very short period of time. Moreover, nearly all of these codes were based on a relatively few ideas about how cities and suburbs ought to be built, meaning that despite the multiplicity of codes there was a remarkable consistency in theme across them. Remaking the country's transportation infrastructure, too, is hardly a new or radical idea: we are emerging from a long period of road-first infrastructure investment that literally changed the country.

We are only a generation or two removed from the most thorough reorganization of space in the history of this country, a reorganization created by a relatively small group of planners, engineers, architects, bureaucrats, reformers, and public health officials who seized upon a small number of ideas and applied them, successfully, right across the country. Robert Moses, the famed planner of New York's public works projects of mid-century, provides a perfect example, having affected change so enormous that even today its scale is difficult to comprehend. The departments under his control, guided by his personal vision of making New York fit for the automobile age, built a dozen expressways (many of which ran straight through existing neighborhoods), ripped up transit lines, constructed enormous bridges and tunnels for cars, re-landscaped a substantial part of New York's environs, and diverted and dammed major rivers. We are not, we should emphasize, calling for methods that would emulate those of Moses (it would be difficult to call his approach to planning "democratic").[8] Yet the example set by Moses and the planners of his generation speaks to the lasting and powerful influence of public policies on the built environment. Even a small reallocation of federal funding away from motorized and toward nonmotorized transportation, to name only one example among many, likely would generate positive results.

To create such change, it is an imperative first step that physical inactivity be treated as highly relevant across a wide variety of fields. The problem of physical activity cannot continue to be viewed in individualistic terms, for solving it will not be accomplished solely through motivating individuals to exercise—modern life is too frazzled, too difficult, and too time-consuming to expect such an approach to work for the majority of people. We must include physical inactivity and poor health among the list of consequences that have accompanied our strategies for building cities, oriented as they have been around a narrow pursuit of largely technocratic goals. We have neglected thousands of years of historical precedent with respect to building healthy, enjoyable, and sustainable places. A major reason why is that we have relegated to the periphery the basic physiological and even psychological need that people have to move under their own power in the built environment. However, major policy tools are in place that can be used effectively to once again support this basic need for "healthy transportation." Many of these same tools can be used to help us design and rebuild healthy, active communities.

Summary of Selected Traffic Calming Studies

Study Locations	Source(s)*	Traffic Calming Measures Taken	Results
Berlin (Germany)	2, 8	Lane narrowings, speed humps, street crossings, plantings, reduction of street space dedicated to cars, speed limitions introduced.	• Increase in street activity by as much as 60 percent • 50 percent increase in bicycle use • Significant accident reductions for most categories of road user
Buxtehude (Germany)	3, 8, 9	Measures included: Tempo 30 zones (reduce average speeds from 50km/h to 30km/h through street redesign measures), street markings to reduce width of driving space, plantings, road humps, traffic islands, road narrowings, and speed-reducing paving design; these were combined with policies to increase walking and bicycling.	• Significant speed reductions • Reduction in noise levels • Significant increases in bicycling • Decreased pedestrian accidents • Decrease in cyclist accident risk
Dortmund (Germany)	8	Tempo 30 measures implemented.	Before-and-after study: • 5.9 percent reduction in cars traveling over 30 km/h • Reductions in numbers of injured pedestrians, including children
France	9	1984–86 program involving 56 local projects. Cycle lanes, pedestrian routes, gate effects, plantings, different paving materials, street redesign.	1987 evaluation found: • 60 percent reduction of serious traffic accidents • Reduction in overall traffic speeds
Gothenburg (Sweden)	2	Creation of traffic cells—five "cells" created in downtown; cars were prevented from crossing the boundaries between cells. Pedestrians, buses, and bicyclists were allowed to do so.	• 45 percent reduction 1970–82 in traffic entering downtown • 50 percent reduction in injury accidents in cells in first 5 years • Decrease in noise and pollution levels

table continues on next page

Study Locations	Source(s)*	Traffic Calming Measures Taken	Results
Groningen (Sweden)	2	Introduction of traffic circulation plan similar to Gothenburg's.	• 44 percent reduction in cars/vans in central area in first year • Increases in walking and bicycling
Hamburg (Germany)	2, 9	Tempo 30 measures implemented.	• 28 percent reduction in traffic fatalities between 1983–1989 in 665 Tempo 30 zones compared to zones where 50 km/h stayed in effect
Hanover (Germany)	2, 9	Reduction of street space dedicated to cars, use of bollards, raised intersections, brick paving, plantings, creation of one-way streets.	• Reduced traffic volume (decrease in through traffic) • Increased use of streets for leisure activities, especially children's play • Increase in length of time people spent on the streets • Increased social interaction
Heidelberg (Germany)	2	Tempo 30 measures implemented.	• 31 percent reduction in accidents • 44 percent reduction in injuries
Nagoya (Japan)	2	Area-wide traffic calming scheme designed to ensure safety and comfort for pedestrians. Followed Osaka experiment.	• Decrease in traffic volumes • Increase in pedestrian and bicycle traffic • Decrease in traffic accidents • Decreased vehicle traffic speeds by 3.5 km/h
International cases (review of comparative findings)	5	Author derived statistics from hundreds of international studies, then assessed how traffic calming measures impact traffic speeds, volumes, and collisions.	• Speed humps had greatest impact on speed reduction, followed by half closures (streets partially shut down to traffic), one-lane slow points, and traffic circles; raised intersections had the least

Study Locations	Source(s)*	Traffic Calming Measures Taken	Results
			• Volume effects greatest when streets fully or half closed, followed by traffic diverters (traffic diverted at intersections); all devices reduced volume on the measured stretch of roadway • All measures substantially reduced collision frequencies in international studies, but less consistent results in United States; author speculates that European countries employ traffic calming devices more intensively than in the U.S., placing multiple devices on a stretch of roadway, leading to increased effects
The Netherlands	2	*Woonerven* routinely used in new residential area design. Substantial street redesign in low-traffic neighborhoods: plantings, obstacles, bottlenecks, benches/play objects, use of varied paving materials, bends in the roadway, restricted access, on-street play areas. *30 km/h zones:* Less ambitious than woonerven. Street design dictates maximum speed of 30 km/h. Speed humps, speed limit signs, street narrowing, parking management, roundabouts. These zones prompted German authorities to create Tempo 30 program.	*Woonerven:* • Reduction in injury accidents by 50 percent • Reported vehicle speeds between 13 and 25 km/h. • Bigger on-street play areas for children considered by residents to be a major benefit • Expensive to create • Strict design requirements not applicable to such as shopping streets or village centers *30 km/h zones:* • 200 zones created in first 3 years of program • First 10 studies showed reductions in vehicle speeds from 27 to 22 km/h, with speed humps and roundabouts the most effective measures

table continues on next page

Study Locations	Source(s)*	Traffic Calming Measures Taken	Results
Odense (Denmark)	7	Project designed to increase safety of children biking/walking to school. Street design changes based on children's identification of dangerous areas. 1981–1990: Of 185 proposals, 65 were accepted. Slow speed areas, road narrowings, traffic islands, separate pedestrian/bicycle paths.	• In slow-speed areas, average speed dropped 30 km/h; reduction in accidents from 9.65/year before changes to 1.5 after • Road narrowings had no effect on accidents, temporary effect on vehicle speed
Osaka (Japan)	2	Creation of "community street." Based on *woonerf* design principles.	• 5 percent increase in pedestrian traffic • 54 percent increase in bicycle traffic • 40 percent decrease in car traffic entering street • Vehicle speeds reduced to between 5 and 8 km/h
Portland, Oregon (United States)	1	Extensive use of traffic circles and speed bumps. Use of entrance treatments, traffic diverters, median barriers, vehicle exclusion lanes, raised crosswalks, pedestrian islands.	• 30 percent reduction in collisions at 8 traffic circles • 36 percent reduction in collisions at 4 speed bumps • Reductions in traffic speed and volume on streets that utilized various calming measures
Seattle (USA)	2	Installation of traffic circles at residential street intersections.	• A study of 14 problem intersections found that the total number collisions dropped from 51.6 to 2.2 after circle installation • A study of 15 intersections found an average reduction from 1.94 to 0.18 collisions per year per location

Study Locations	Source(s)*	Traffic Calming Measures Taken	Results
Skaerbaek (Denmark)	2	Package of measures designed to reduce speed of through traffic on main road. Also, creation of cycle paths.	• Increase in the percentage of people indicating ease of movement throughout town • Reduction in car speeds from 58 to 51 kmh and large truck speeds from 55 to 46 km/h
United States (multiple cities)	6	Study of traffic calming devices (bulbouts, raised crosswalks, raised intersections, refuge islands) installed in multiple cities around the United States.	• Inconsistent results with respect to effects on vehicle speeds, pedestrian use of crosswalks, pedestrian wait time, other motorist behavior • Study employed devices singly—no attempt to understand the effects of combinations of devices over the same stretch of roadway
Vancouver (Canada)	10	Four projects reviewed by author: Projects involved street closures, diagonal diverters, traffic circles, one-way streets, street closures, build-outs, speed humps, build-outs, stop signs.	• All four projects experienced reductions in collision frequency, severity, and annual collision claim costs. Collision frequency fell between 18 and 60 percent; annual claim costs fell between 10 and 57 percent.

*. 1. City of Portland, Oregon, Office of Transportation (1999), "Collisions on Traffic Calmed Streets," "Portland Project Evaluations," at www.trans.ci.portland.or.us. 2. Clark & Dornfeld (1994), *National Bicycling and Walking Study; FHWA Case Study No. 19: Traffic Calming, Auto-Restricted Zones and Other Traffic Management Techniques—Their Effects on Bicycling and Pedestrians.* 3. Doldissen and Draeger (1993), "Environmental traffic management strategies in Buxtehude, West Germany," in Rodney Tolley (ed.), *The Greening of Urban Transport.* 4. Eubank-Ahrens (1987), "A Closer Look at the Users of Woonerven," in Anne Vernez Moudon (ed.), *Public Streets for Public Use.* 5. Ewing, Reid (2001), "Impacts of Traffic Calming," *Transportation Quarterly* 55. 6. Federal Highway Administration (2000), *The Effects of Traffic Calming Measures on Pedestrian and Motorist Behavior.* 7. Nielson (1993), "Safe routes to school in Odense, Denmark," in Tolley (1993). 8. Whitelegg (1993), "The principle of environmental traffic management," in Tolley (1993). 9. Wynne (1992), *A Study of Bicycle and Pedestrian Programs in European Countries.* 10. Zein et al. (1997), "Safety Benefits of Traffic Calming," *Transportation Research Record:* 1578.

CHAPTER 2

1. Historians argue that the suburban ideal was firmly established in the minds of developers, architects, housing reformers, and others by the end of World War I, a development partly influenced by the unhealthy living conditions in the central city of the nineteenth century. See Jackson 1985, Sies 1987.

2. The essay quoted is Olmsted, Vaux and Company, "Observations on the Progress of Improvements in Street Plans, with Special Reference to the Parkway Proposed to Be Laid out in Brooklyn," Brooklyn, 1868. Contained in Sutton 1971.

3. In his "Report to the Staten Island Improvement Commission of a Preliminary Scheme for Improvements," Olmsted included the transcript of an interview between himself and Elisha Harris on the subject of the causes and prevention of malaria on the island. Harris stated that malaria is "a poison in the atmosphere." The poisonous atmospheres, Harris argued, are found near marshes and other low-lying, damp ground. In contrast, trees and other plants were viewed as having a beneficial effect in countering diseases such as malaria; malarial "spores or germs would be arrested by and fasten to the foliage." Moreover, trees and tree belts would have additional benefits by soaking up moisture in the soil. See Fein 1967, 207–37. See also the summary of this interview in Szczygiel and Hewitt 2000.

4. Quotation from Olmsted et al., "Report to the Staten Island Improvement Commission of a Preliminary Scheme for Improvements" (1871) in Fein 1967.

5. First quotation from Olmsted and Vaux, "Preliminary Report to the Commissioners for Laying Out a Park in Brooklyn, New York: Being a Consideration of Circumstances of Site and Other Conditions Affecting the Design of Public Pleasure Grounds" (1866), in Fein 1967. Second quotation from Olmsted, Vaux and Company, "Preliminary Report upon the Proposed Suburban Village at Riverside, near Chicago" (1868), in Sutton 1971.

6. During the middle of the nineteenth century, the period in which the sanitation reform movement was born, the miasmatic position was by far the more important theory. During this period, however, there was some movement to combine the miasmatic and contagionist positions into a single theory. See Szczygiel and Hewitt 2000.

7. Charles Chapin, Superintendent of Health for Providence, Rhode Island, gave a presentation in 1902 to the annual meeting of the American Public Health Administration, at which he stated, "municipal cleanliness does little to prevent

infection or decrease the death rate. I would plead with health officers for a more rational perspective in directing their efforts and to devote more attention to the isolation of infectious diseases . . . [and] pay a little less attention to finical defects in plumbing, to stable manure and garbage buckets." See Charles Chapin, "Dirt, Disease, and the Health Officer," in American Public Health Association 1977, 296–9.

8. In American Public Health Association 1977, see especially Lawrence Flick, "The Essentials in the Crusade Against Tuberculosis," 128–35.

9. See Lubove 1967; Veiller 1929, 1970. Veiller was unoriginal in this respect— the need for more and better "light and air" was commonly expressed in housing, planning, and architectural circles during this period. Architects and engineers had begun to make systematic studies of sunlight and shadow on building size, location, and design. Boston architect William Atkinson, who focused on how to orient buildings to maximize sunlight, did the first in 1912. He stated that health considerations were the major basis for this work, a position no doubt influenced by his professional experience as a designer of hospitals. See Atkinson 1912. See also the later study on the same subject, by Heydecker and Goodrich (1929).

10. The two-volume report issued by the Tenement House Commission included physicians' reports testifying to the closeness of the relationship between light, air, and tuberculosis on the one hand, and the incidence of tuberculosis and the tenement on the other. See for example Biggs 1903, Guerard 1903.

11. Marcuse (1977) asserted that early city planners sought to protect the financial security of the middle and upper classes (through the protection of real estate values). Housing for the poor was not an important part of their agenda. Likewise, historical research by Weiss (1987) of zoning in Los Angeles revealed that the early stages of zoning were animated by a desire, on behalf of influential members of the real estate industry, to protect high-income neighborhoods from intrusion by unwanted groups. Only later (1930s) were middle-class neighborhoods viewed as worthy of zoning protection. There were, of course, exceptions to the general thesis that the suburb was desirable only to those who wanted to profit from their construction: some, like the members of the Regional Planning Association of America, wanted to build suburban enclaves containing good housing for lower-income groups.

12. Zoning's appeal extended to many who were involved in housing reform issues in the first two decades of the century. Many coupled the promise of low-cost land in suburban areas with affordable low-density housing—the key was to first develop and then protect over time those neighborhoods that possessed such attributes. See the discussion in Spann (1996) of the architects Charles Whitaker and Frederick Ackerman, members of the Regional Planning Association of

America; Ackerman saw the potential inherent in zoning, but also lamented the likelihood that it would be used for exclusionary purposes.

13. The book's original title was *Tomorrow: A Peaceful Path to Real Reform,* published in 1898. It was reissued in 1902 under the name *Garden Cities of Tomorrow,* which is the version that made Howard famous.

14. A consensus position within planning had emerged by 1920 that asserted that the automobile would be good for cities, chiefly by enabling the dispersion of the population to outlying suburbs, thereby improving congestion in the inner city. See Foster 1981, chapter 5.

15. See for example the series of essays in a volume published in 1958 by the editors of *Fortune* magazine (titled *The Exploding Metropolis*). Whyte railed against sprawl while Jacobs attacked urban renewal projects in the inner cities. Whyte's essay, in particular, eerily presaged contemporary debate on the causes and consequences of urban growth. "Sprawl," he wrote, "is bad aesthetics; it is bad economics. Five acres are being made to do the work of one, and do it very poorly. This is bad for the farmers, it is bad for communities, it is bad for the railroads, it is bad for the recreation groups, it is bad even for the developers. And it is unnecessary. In many suburbs the opportunity has vanished, but it is not too late to lay down sensible guidelines for the communities of the future" (Editors of *Fortune* magazine 1958, 134–135).

CHAPTER 3

1. The determination of one's weight status is defined by public health agencies using a measure called body mass index (BMI), which is a ratio of a person's weight to their height. The CDC defines a healthy BMI for an adult at 18–25 kilograms per square meter (kg/m^2). An overweight person is defined as having a BMI of 25–29.9 kg/m^2 while someone who is defined as obese has a BMI of 30 kg/m^2 and over.

2. This is also the position taken by the Centers for Disease Control. See "Obesity and Overweight: A Public Health Epidemic." Available online at http://cdc.gov/nccdphp/dnpa/obesity/epidemic.htm.

CHAPTER 4

1. Unfortunately, the data that was collected in Seattle did not contain information specific to parks, making more precise linkages between neighborhood age, location of parks, and travel behavior impossible. An additional problem stems from the simple observation that the oldest parts of most regions also happen to be located closer to the region's core, where there are more recreational attractions; the relationship between age of development and travel to recreational destinations may therefore be a proxy for regional location.

2. In 2002, the *American Journal of Preventive Medicine* reported the findings of a study that showed that American adults who lived in older homes were significantly more likely to walk than those who lived in newer homes (homes were a proxy for the age of development in the surrounding area). In this study, people in newer homes (built after 1973) were less likely to walk one or more miles per month (and at least twenty times per month) than people who lived in homes built before 1973. See Berrigan and Troiano 2002.

3. The NPTS draws from large samples of the civilian, noninstitutionalized population of the United States aged five and older and collects information on all trips, mode share, trip purposes, and travel in urban and rural areas. The NPTS was conducted in 1969, 1977, 1983, 1990, 1995 and 2001 (under a different name).

4. According to the 1995 NPTS, of the walk trips, 77 percent were for personal or social purposes, 14 percent were to church or school, and 7 percent were to work. Of the bike trips, personal and recreational travel accounted for 82 percent, church and school 9 percent, and work 8 percent (FHWA 1997).

5. This survey also found that nearly one in five respondents were female. The geographical location within the region from which these data were drawn may have influenced the findings. Moritz drew his data from a trail that is used exclusively by walkers, cyclists, and other nonmotorized users. Many studies of bicycling gather data from such trails.

6. It is important to note that the set of nations shown here is not intended to be representative of all countries around the globe.

7. See the website of the Congress for New Urbanism, the leading organization dedicated to New Urbanism, at www.cnu.org.

CHAPTER 5

1. The referenced data is provided by the Youth Risk Behavior Surveillance System (YRBSS), a comprehensive system of surveys conducted by the Centers for Disease Control as well as state and local health agencies. The referenced statistics can be found in Grunbaum et al. 2002, table 40.

2. Percentages total to more than 100 percent because respondents were given the choice to indicate more than one barrier.

3. The findings concerning the basic spatial attributes of German cities are consistent with those made by other scholars of that country's transportation systems and land use patterns. For further discussion, see chapters 7 and 9.

4. This phenomenon is not limited to the United States. A Japanese study conducted in 1990, for example, found a significant correlation between walking speed and age, especially for those over seventy-five years of age, whose walking speed was only 72 percent of the speed of adults aged nineteen to thirty-five; when this walking speed was compared with the green-light time of pedestrian signals

in Japan, crossing times were inadequate for the speed at which the elderly walk. See OECD 1998.

5. The referenced study is known by the acronym SMARTRAQ, short for *Strategies for Metropolitan Atlanta's Regional Transportation and Air Quality.* SMARTRAQ is a regional transportation and land use study and includes a component aimed at better understanding the physical activity patterns in the built environment. SMARTRAQ is funded by a consortium of agencies, including the Georgia Department of Transportation, Georgia Regional Transportation Authority, Centers for Disease Control and Prevention, The Turner Foundation, and the Environmental Protection Agency. See www.smartraq.net.

6. MARTA stands for Metropolitan Atlanta Rapid Transit Authority.

CHAPTER 6

1. In *A Pattern Language,* architect Christopher Alexander and his co-authors made an important contribution to understanding the hundreds of ways that the built environment can be designed so as to create more humane and livable cities. All attributes of the environment, Alexander insists, from the larger pieces such as entire transportation systems down to the smallest pieces within individual buildings, are necessarily linked; failure to plan and build with this in mind will result in environments that do not function as intended. "When you build a thing you cannot merely build the thing in isolation, but must also repair the world around it, and within it, so that the larger world at that one place becomes more coherent, and more whole" (Alexander et al. 1977, xiii).

2. This calculation is derived from data produced by the SMARTRAQ study in Atlanta (see endnote 5, chapter 5). Only about one-half of a percent of one-kilometer squares laid over metropolitan Atlanta (a thirteen-county region) consisted of both relatively high proximity (high net residential density) *and* connectivity (high street intersection density, consisting of the number of inter-sections within the square kilometer). Therefore, the great majority of one-kilometer squares in this thirteen-county area (over 10,000 such squares) did not meet both the proximity and connectivity thresholds set by this analysis. More information about SMARTRAQ can be found at www.smartraq.net.

3. The data source for this finding is the SMARTRAQ study.

CHAPTER 7

1. Perry clearly wanted to make auto travel within the neighborhood as dffiicult as possible: "If in the process of highway specialization we adapt park-ways and boulevards to the needs of vehicles, why should we not fit neighborhood streets to the special requirements of pedestrians? . . . Suppose the residential streets do seem like a labyrinth, and some of them are so narrow that, with cars

parked at the curb, passage for other cars is a slow process—are not the safety and tranquillity (sic) thus obtained worth more than the convenience that is sacrificed?" (Perry 1939, 56, 74).

2. Statistics are available on-line at http://www.railtrails.org. Accessed March 25, 2002.

3. The linkage between transit and walking is an old idea and a well-researched phenomenon. A study by Cervero and Radisch (1995), for example, studied the relationship between traditional neighborhood design and transit demand in the San Francisco Bay area. In the community with higher density levels, transit and walking both benefited from higher density levels. Transit ridership levels and levels of walking and biking were greater for both work and non-work trips in the community that had higher density levels.

CHAPTER 8

1. For a contrary position see the discussion on Randall Crane's research in chapter 6.

2. In Atlanta, for example, many of the city's wealthy, older neighborhoods contain well-constructed apartment buildings that exist harmoniously alongside single-family dwellings. These neighborhoods, including Inman Park, Virginia Highlands, Midtown, Ansley Park, Ponce Highlands, and Candler Park, are now considered to be among the most desirable in the city, with housing prices well above the median price for homes in the region. Similar observations can be made for cities around the country, especially those that have shared in the widespread urban renaissance that began in the United States in the late 1980s and early 1990s.

CHAPTER 9

1. The information in table 9-1 is provided by a review conducted by transportation planner Reid Ewing (Ewing 1994). Ewing compared American, British, and Australian residential street design guidelines, using standards contained in authoritative manuals in each country, and found that minimum road widths and turning radii were significantly larger in the American manual than in the British and Australian cases (turning radii are larger to extend sight distances for motorists, resulting in higher turning speeds). Along those streets where the British and Australian standards did not require sidewalks, both manuals mandated the use of intensive traffic calming methods and other design features to ensure that traffic could not safely move at speeds faster than twenty miles per hour.

2. Applying numbers to terms such as "uncomfortably crowded" or "overcrowded" would be exceedingly difficult, as crowding is an inherently subjective

experience. Not only does the definition of overcrowding vary from person to person, each individual's assessment of overcrowding can vary from place to place. Also, different cultural settings likely produce different reactions with respect to what differentiates a comfortable experience from an uncomfortable one. For a fuller exposition see Churchman 1999.

3. Raised crosswalks have the potential to be safer than crosswalks that are placed on the same level as the carriageway. In *A Pattern Language*, Christopher Alexander and co-authors write, "No amount of painted white lines, crosswalks, traffic lights, button operated signals, ever quite manage to change the fact that a car weighs a ton or more, and will run over any pedestrian, unless the driver brakes. . . . The people who cross a road will only feel comfortable and safe if the road crossing is a physical obstruction, which physically guarantees that the cars must slow down and give way to pedestrians." See Alexander et al. 1977, 281.

4. In a 1997 article in *Governing* magazine, Alan Ehrenhalt wrote that ITE is a more progressive rival to AASHTO because it has a broader constituency, consisting of planners and consultants as well as engineers. See Ehrenhalt 1997.

CHAPTER 10

1. Figure 10-4 references "net" residential density as the unit of measurement for density. This term is important because it conveys that the measurement was based on the number of households per land area that is in residential use in the area in which the household is located. As referenced in chapter 5, the Atlanta region has one of the lowest population densities in the United States; this is reflected in the study design, where the highest level of density began at 8 dwelling units per acre, a number that would be considered very low in many other regions, especially abroad. Additionally, it is important to note that the findings reported here reflect results for SMARTRAQ survey respondents; the SMARTRAQ survey was designed to include a slightly higher percentage of respondents from higher-density neighborhoods so as to ensure that enough data would be available from such neighborhoods for statistical analysis.

CHAPTER 11

1. For a discussion of these problems, see Beaumont and Pianca 2000.

2. Pietro Nivola, a Brookings Institution fellow, estimates that between 1977 and 1995, all levels of government in the United States spent $1.2 *trillion* on roads and highways, $0.2 trillion on mass transit and $13 billion on intercity passenger rail (Amtrak)—meaning that transit spending was a sixth that of highways and passenger rail was a hundredth as much. The federal government controls a large share of this funding, sending much of it directly to the states. See Nivola 1999.

3. ISTEA stands for Intermodal Surface Transportation Act. TEA-21 stands for Transportation Equity Act for the twenty-first Century.

4. For further discussion of these issues, see Surface Transportation Policy Project *Changing Direction: Federal Transportation Spending in the 1990s* (April 2000). Available at http://www.transact.org.

5. Georgia's Environmental Protection Division estimates that half of the Atlanta region's output of nitrogen oxide (NO_x, an ozone precursor) is produced by automobiles and trucks, while only a bit over 20 percent comes from point sources. See *Georgia's Environment*, April 2001, available at www.state.ga.us/dnr/environ.

6. This claim is not meant to imply that New Urbanists and smart growth advocates have failed to address these issues. As illustrated in Calthorpe (1993) and Duany and Talen (2002), New Urbanists are aware of systematic problems that hinder or prohibit altogether the creation of a built environment that comprehensively address regional problems. Calthorpe addresses transit provision while Duany and Talen address zoning codes.

7. See, e.g., report by Jack Faucett Associates and Sierra Research, Inc., 1999, *Granting Air Quality Credit for Land Use Measures: Policy Options*, Prepared for the U.S. Environmental Protection Agency, September 8, 1999, Report No. SR99-09-01.

8. In his biography of Robert Moses, *The Power Broker*, Robert Caro details the brute force approach to planning of Moses and the city departments under him, an approach which worked well for the brilliant and charismatic Moses until the 1960s, when enough serious objections began to slow the furious pace of his construction agenda; among others, Jane Jacobs was involved in fights with Moses during this period to stop his highways from destroying neighborhoods in Manhattan. See Caro 1975.

Body Mass Index (BMI):   A measure used to assess the weight status of individuals. It is a ratio of a person's weight to their height. Public health agencies have defined a healthy BMI for an adult at 18–25 kilograms per square meter (kg/m^2).

Built environment: A term referring to the physical form and character of communities. In the model presented in this book, the built environment consists of three elements—transportation systems, land use patterns, and urban design characteristics.

Carriageway: Street lanes dedicated to moving traffic.

Chronic disease: Illnesses that are prolonged, have multiple causes (frequently having to do with behavioral patterns), do not resolve spontaneously, and are rarely cured completely.

Connectivity: A term describing how directly a person can travel from one destination to another via existing transportation networks.

Density: Term referring to the concentration of people, objects, or trip ends within the built environment. Density influences proximity.

Duration (of exercise):   The length of time needed to engage in a particular type of physical activity.

Employment density: A measure of density indicating the concentration of employees within a given geographic area.

Exercise: Structured physical activity, usually vigorous, that is done during leisure time for purposes of physical fitness.

Facade: The design features of the front of a building—its architectural style, door and window treatments, portico, stoop, texture, and so on.

Grid, modified grid networks: High-connectivity street networks based on a formal, perpendicular arrangement of streets.

Hierarchical networks: Low-connectivity street networks wherein streets are ordered into a hierarchy, based upon traffic movement. At the top are arterial roads, designed for high-volume automobile traffic. At the bottom are local residential streets, designed for a low volume of automobile through traffic.

Infectious disease: A synonym for communicable disease. An illness due to an infectious agent that arises through direct transmission from an infected person, animal, or other source to a host or indirectly through an intermediate source.

Intensity (of exercise): The level of energy required of physical activity.

Land use patterns: Consist of the spatial arrangement of structures and other physical elements within the built environment. Determine how close destinations are to one another (proximity).

Metabolic equivalent (MET): A measure of the oxygen consumption required for physical activity. One MET equates to $(3.5 \text{ ml O}^2) / (\text{kg/min})$, which is the metabolic rate of a person at rest.

Mixed-use development: Land-use development wherein different types of uses (e.g., commercial and residential) are located within close proximity to one another.

Mode share: The share, by percentage, of trips by each type of mode (e.g., automobile, transit, walking, bicycling).

Moderate physical activity: A type of physical activity defined by public health agencies as requiring 3 to 6 metabolic equivalents (METs), which is the amount of energy required for the heart to work at 50 percent to 69 percent of its maximum rate (see USDHHS 1999).

Neighborhood grain: The size and texture of structures and other basic elements within a neighborhood.

Neo-traditional design: A term referring to urban design theories and techniques that emphasize the virtues of older neighborhoods: a fine neighborhood grain, grid street patterns, human-scaled architecture, a mixture of uses.

New Urbanism: A term describing an architect-led movement based on neo-traditional design principles.

Obesity: A person is classified by public health agencies as being obese if their body mass index (BMI) is 30 or over.

Organic networks: High-connectivity street networks formed as a result of gradual changes over many decades or centuries. Typically found in the oldest parts of old cities. Streets extend in all directions, exhibiting little or no formal pattern. Highly walkable.

Overweight: A person is classified by public health agencies as being over-weight if their body mass index (BMI) is between 25 and 29.9.

Parking lane: A lane on the street that consists of parked cars. Located in between the carriageway and the sidewalk.

Physical activity: Movement of the body's muscles requiring an expenditure of energy above 1 metabolic equivalent.

Physically inactive: A term describing a person who gets little or no physical activity.

Population density: A measure of density indicating the number of people within a given geographic area.

Proximity: The crow-fly distance between two destinations.

Recreational physical activity: Physical activity that is undertaken during one's leisure hours. Is usually nonpurposive.

Residential density: A measure of density indicating the number of residents within a given geographic area.

Sedentary: A term describing a completely inactive lifestyle.

Setback: The distance between a building's facade and the street. Conventional zoning codes typically mandate large setbacks to accommodate parking in front of commercial structures.

Single-use development: Development wherein land use types (e.g., commercial, residential, industrial) are kept separate from one another.

Site design: The design elements of a site (e.g., a plot of land on which a building sits) that are believed to influence a person's desire to walk or bicycle.

Specialized networks: Facilities that are not a part of either the street surface or the area immediately adjacent to the street and that are dedicated to nonmotorized travel and physical activity. Include specialized bicycle facilities, shared facilities that accommodate multiple uses (trails for bicyclists, joggers, etc.), and pedestrian paths that link in-town destinations.

Street design: General term referencing design strategies that make streets more amenable for motorized or nonmotorized transportation.

Street furniture: Objects on the sidewalk such as benches, lampposts, trees, and mailboxes.

Street networks: Street networks provide links between places for different modes of travel (light rail and bus transit, automobile, bicycle, pedestrian). They influence how far one has to travel to reach a destination as well as how many route options one has to choose from.

Street trees: Trees planted immediately adjacent to the street surface (carriageway or parking lane).

Traffic calming: Term for strategies that attempt to slow motorized traffic and enhance nonmotorized travel through street redesign. Strategies include placing humps, plantings, and other objects in the carriageway, narrowing the width of the street at key points such as pedestrian crossings, and other similar measures.

Transit systems: Bus and rail systems that may or may not operate along the street network. Are relevant to discussion on physical activity because, when designed properly, such systems give pedestrians and, to a lesser extent, bicyclists more capacity for moving about in the built environment without needing an automobile.

Transit-Oriented Development (TOD): A type of development that surrounds a transit stop with a mixture of uses (e.g., housing, shopping, and office space), high population densities, and pedestrian-oriented design.

Transportation systems: Transportation systems connect places to each other. They influence how easy or difficult it is to use different types of transportation to get from one place to another. Different transportation systems include streets and roads, transit systems, and specialized networks.

Trip-end density: A measure of density indicating the number of trip ends (basically, the origin or destination of a trip) within a given geographic area.

Urban design: Term describing the design and styling of buildings, streets, and other elements of the built environment.

Urban form: A general term referring to the spatial arrangement and layout of objects and networks within cities, towns, and suburbs.

Utilitarian physical activity: Physical activity that is undertaken as a consequence of doing other things (e.g., working, shopping, traveling).

Vertical integration: Mixed-use development wherein uses are mixed within the same structure. The most common example is a building containing retail on the ground floor and apartments on the upper floors.

Vigorous physical activity: A type of physical activity defined by public health agencies as requiring more than 6 METs, which is the amount of energy required for the heart to work at greater than 70 percent of its maximum rate (see USDHHS 1999).

Walkable environment: Neighborhoods or districts that encourage walking by containing multiple attributes: wide sidewalks, provision of "street furniture," short building setbacks, well-marked and frequent crosswalks, traffic calming, high residential and commercial densities, mixed uses, and public amenities such as squares, parks, and other gathering places.

Woonerf: Dutch term describing a radical form of traffic calming, wherein the object is to reduce motorized traffic speed to perhaps seven miles per hour and to turn the street into a social space for people who are not in vehicles.

Alexander, Christopher, Sara Ishikawa, and Murray Silverstein with Max Jacobson, Ingrid Fiksdahl-King, and Shlomo Angel. 1977. *A Pattern Language: Towns, Buildings, Construction*. New York: Oxford University Press.

Allen, Irving. 1977. New towns and the suburban dream. In Irving Allen (Ed.), *New Towns and the Suburban Dream: Ideology and Utopia in Planning and Development*. Port Washington, NY: Kennikat Press.

American Public Health Association. 1977. *Selections from Public Health Reports and Papers Presented at the Meetings of the American Public Health Association (1884–1907)*. New York: Arno Press.

————. 1948. *Planning the Neighborhood*. American Public Health Association, Committee on the Hygiene of Housing. Chicago: Public Administration Service.

Andersen, Ross, Thomas Wadden, Susan Bartlett, Babette Zemel, Tony Verde, and Shawn Franckowiak. 1999. Effects of lifestyle activity versus structured aerobic exercise in obese women. *Journal of the American Medical Association* 281: 335–40.

Antonakos, Cathy. 1995. Nonmotor travel in the 1990 Nationwide Personal Transportation Survey. *Transportation Research Record* 1502: 75–81.

————. 1994. Environmental and travel preferences of cyclists. *Transportation Research Record* 1438: 75–81.

Antupit, Stephen, Barbara Gray, and Sandra Woods. 1996. Steps ahead: making streets that work in Seattle, Washington. *Landscape and Urban Planning* 35: 107–22.

Apogee Research, Inc. 1998. *The Effects of Urban Form on Travel and Emissions: A Review and Synthesis of the Literature*. Washington, D.C.: Draft report prepared for the United States Environmental Protection Agency. HBIX Reference C611-005.

Appleyard, Donald. 1981. *Livable Streets*. Berkeley: University of California Press.

Appleyard. Donald and Mark Lintell. 1982. The environmental quality of city streets: The residents' viewpoint. In Stephen Kaplan and Rachel Kaplan (Eds.), *Humanscape: Environments for People*. Ann Arbor, MI: Ulrich's Books, Inc.

Atkinson, William. 1912. *The Orientation of Buildings or Planning for Sunlight*. New York: John Wiley and Sons.

Balfour, Jennifer and George Kaplan. 2002. Neighborhood environment and loss of physical function in older adults: evidence from the Alameda County Study. *American Journal of Epidemiology* 155: 507–15.

Ball, Kylie, Adrian Bauman, Eva Leslie, and Neville Owen. 2001. Perceived environmental aesthetics and convenience and company are associated with walking for exercise among Australian adults. *Preventive Medicine* 33: 434–40.

Bassett, Edward. 1925. Zoning roundtable. *City Planning* 1, 1: 60–1 (April 1925).

Beatley, Timothy. 2000. *Green Urbanism: Learning from European Cities.* Washington, D.C.: Island Press.

Beaumont, Constance and Elizabeth Pianca. 2000. *Historic Neighborhoods in the Age of Sprawl: Why Johnny Can't Walk to School.* Washington, D.C.: National Trust for Historic Preservation. Available on-line at www.nationaltrust.org.

Berrigan, David and Richard Troiano. 2002. The association between urban form and physical activity in the United States. *American Journal of Preventive Medicine* 23, 2, Supplement 1: 74–9.

Beuscher, Jacob, Robert Wright, and Morton Gitelman. 1976. *Cases and Materials on Land Use.* American Casebook Series. Second Edition. St. Paul, MN: West Publishing Co.

Beyard, Michael and Michael Pawlukiewicz. 2001. *Ten Principles for Reinventing America's Suburban Strips.* Washington, D.C.: ULI—Urban Land Institute.

Biggs, Herman. 1903. Tuberculosis and the Tenement House Problem. In Robert DeForest and Lawrence Veiller (Eds.), *The Tenement House Problem, Including the Report of the New York State Tenement House Commission of 1900.* Volume one (two volumes). New York: The Macmillan Company.

Blair, Steven, Harold Kohl, Ralph Paffenbarger, Diane Clark, K. Cooper, and L. Gibbons. 1989. Physical fitness and all-cause mortality: a prospective study of healthy men and women. *Journal of the American Medical Association* 273: 1093–8.

Booth, Michael, Adrian Bauman, Neville Owen, and Christopher Gore. 1997. Physical activity preferences, preferred sources of assistance, and perceived barriers to increased activity among physically inactive Australians. *Preventive Medicine* 26: 131–7.

Bouchard, Claude, and Roy Shephard. 1994. *Physical activity, fitness, and health: International proceedings and consensus statement.* Conference Proceedings. Champaign, IL: Human Kinetics Publishers.

Brieger, Gert. 1978. Sanitary reform in New York City: Stephen Smith and the passage of the Metropolitan Health Bill. In John Leavitt and Ronald Numbers (Eds.), *Sickness and Health in America: Readings in the History of Medicine and Public Health.* Madison, WI: The University of Wisconsin Press.

Brooks, Arthur. 1989. The office file box—Emanations from the battlefield. In Charles Haar and Jerold Kayden (Eds.), *Zoning and the American Dream: Promises Still to Keep.* Chicago: Planners Press, American Planning Association.

Brownson, Ross, Elizabeth Baker, Robyn Housemann, Laura Brennan, and

Stephen Bacak. 2001. Environmental and policy determinants of physical activity in the United States. *American Journal of Public Health* 91, 12: 1995–2003.

Buder, Stanley. 1990. *Visionaries and Planners: The Garden City Movement and the Modern Community.* New York: Oxford University Press.

Bullard, Robert, Glenn Johnson, and Angel Torres. 1999. *Sprawl Atlanta: Social Equity Dimensions of Uneven Growth and Development.* Atlanta, GA: Clark Atlanta University, Environmental Justice Resource Center.

Burrington, Stephen. 1996. Restoring the rule of law and respect for communities in transportation. *New York University Environmental Law Journal* 5: 691–734.

Calthorpe, Peter. 1993. *The Next American Metropolis: Ecology, Community, and the American Dream.* New York: Princeton Architectural Press.

Caro, Robert. 1975. *The Power Broker: Robert Moses and the Fall of New York.* New York: Vintage Books.

Centers for Disease Control and Prevention. 2002a. Barriers to children walking and biking to school—United States, 1999. *Morbidity and Mortality Weekly Report* 51, 32: 701–4.

———. 2002b. School transportation modes—Georgia, 2000. *Morbidity and Mortality Weekly Report* 51, 32: 704–5.

———. 2001a. Increasing physical activity: a report on recommendations of the Task Force on Community Preventive Services. *Morbidity and Mortality Weekly Report* 50, RR18: 1–16.

———. 2001b. Physical Activity Trends—United States, 1990–1998. *Morbidity and Mortality Weekly Report* 50, 9: 166–9.

———. 1999a. *Chronic Diseases and Their Risk Factors: The Nation's Leading Causes of Death.* Atlanta: Centers for Disease Control and Prevention.

———. 1999b. Neighborhood safety and the prevalence of physical inactivity—selected states, 1996. *Morbidity and Mortality Weekly Report* 48, 7: 143–6.

———. 1999c. Pedestrian fatalities—Cobb, DeKalb, Fulton, and Gwinnett Counties, Georgia, 1994–1998. *Morbidity and Mortality Weekly Report* 48, 28: 601–5.

———. 1999d. Prevalence of overweight among children and adolescents: United States, 1999. Hyattsville, MD: National Center for Health Statistics. Available on-line at: www.cdc.gov/nchs/products/pubs/pubd/hestats/over99fig1.htm.

———. 1990. Coronary heart disease attributable to sedentary lifestyle—selected states, 1988. *Morbidity and Mortality Weekly Report* 39: 541–4.

Cervero, Robert. 1991. Congestion relief: the land use alternative. *Journal of Planning, Education and Research* 10: 119–29.

———. 1988. Land-use mixing and suburban mobility. *Transportation Quarterly* 42, 3: 429–46.

————. 1986. *Suburban Gridlock.* New Brunswick, N.J.: Center for Urban Policy Research.

Cervero, Robert and Carolyn Radisch. 1995. *Travel Choices in Pedestrian versus Automobile Oriented Neighborhoods.* Working Paper 644. University of California at Berkeley. Berkeley, CA: Institute of Urban and Regional Development.

Christensen, Carol. 1986. *The American Garden City and the New Towns Movement.* Ann Arbor, MI: UMI Research Press.

Churchman, Arza. 1999. Disentangling the concept of density. *Journal of Planning Literature* 13, 4: 389–411.

City of Portland, Oregon. 1999. *Collisions on traffic calmed streets.* Available on-line at www.trans.ci.portland.or.us/Traff...ent/Trafficcalming/reports/accidents.html. Portland, OR: Office of Transportation.

Clarke, Andrew and Michael Dornfeld. 1994. *National Bicycling and Walking Study, FHWA Case Study No. 19: Traffic Calming, Auto-Restricted Zones and Other Traffic Management Techniques—Their Effects on Bicycling and Pedestrians.* Washington, D.C.: Federal Highway Administration.

Corbett, Judith and Joe Velasquez. 1994. *The Ahwahnee Principles: Toward More Livable Communities.* Sacramento: Center for Livable Communities.

Coughlin, Joseph. 2001. *Transportation and Older Persons: Perceptions and Preferences, A Report on Focus Groups.* Washington, D.C.: American Association of Retired Persons. Available on-line at http://research.aarp.org/ il/2001_05_transport.pdf.

Coughlin, Joseph and Annalynn Lacombe. 1997. Ten myths about transportation for the elderly. *Transportation Quarterly* 51, 1: 91–100.

Craig, Cora, Ross Brownson, Sue Cragg, and Andrea Dunn. 2002. Exploring the effect of the environment on physical activity: a study examining walking to work. *American Journal of Preventive Medicine* 23, 2, Supplement 1: 36–43.

Crane, Randall. 1999. *The Impacts of Urban Form on Travel: A Critical Review.* Cambridge, Mass.: Lincoln Institute of Land Policy Working Paper No. WP99RC1.

————. 1996a. Cars and drivers in the new suburbs: linking access to travel in neo-traditional planning. *Journal of the American Planning Association* 62, 1: 51–63.

————. 1996b. On form versus function: will the New Urbanism reduce traffic, or increase it? *Journal of Planning Education and Research* 15: 117–26.

Daisa, Jim, Michael Jones, and Alan Wachtel. 1996. Children, traffic and safety: responding to the school commute. *Institute of Transportation Engineers 66th Annual Meeting: 1996 Compendium of Technical Papers*: 163–6.

Davis, Adrian. 1998. Walking and safer routes to school. *Traffic Engineering and Control* (March): 171–3.

DeForest, Robert and Lawrence Veiller. 1903. The tenement house problem. In Robert DeForest and Lawrence Veiller (Eds.), *The Tenement House Problem, Including the Report of the New York State Tenement House Commission of 1900.* Volume one (2 volumes). New York: The Macmillan Company.

Derby, C., B. Mohr, I. Goldstein, H. Feldman, C. Johannes, and J. McKinlay. 2000. Modifiable risk factors and erectile dysfunction: can lifestyle changes modify risk? *Urology* 56, 2: 302–6.

Dixon, Linda. 1995. Bicycle and pedestrian level-of-service performance measures and standards for congestion management systems. *Transportation Research Record* 1538: 1–9.

Döldissen, Alice, and Werner Draeger. 1993. Environmental traffic management strategies in Buxtehude, West Germany. In Rodney Tolley (ed.), *The Greening of Urban Transport: Planning for Walking and Cycling in Western Cities.* London: Belhaven Press.

Duany, Andres, and Emily Talen. 2002. Transect planning. *Journal of the American Planning Association* 68, 3: 245–66.

Duffy, John. 1978. Social impact of disease in the late nineteenth century. In John Leavitt and Ronald Numbers (Eds.), *Sickness and Health in America: Readings in the History of Medicine and Public Health.* Madison, WI: The University of Wisconsin Press.

———. 1968. *A History of Public Health in New York City 1625–1866.* New York: Russell Sage Foundation.

Dunn, Andrea, Ross Andersen, and John Jakicic. 1998. Lifestyle physical activity interventions: history, short- and long-term effects, and recommendations. *American Journal of Preventive Medicine* 15, 4: 398–412.

Dunn, Andrea, Melissa Garcia, Bess Marcus, James Kampert, Harold Kohl, and Steven Blair. 1998. Six-month physical activity and fitness changes in Project Active, a randomized trial. *Medicine and Science in Sports and Exercise* 30, 7: 1076–83.

Dunn, Andrea, Bess Marcus, James Kampert, Melissa Garcia, Harold Kohl, and Steven Blair. 1999. Comparison of lifestyle and structured interventions to increase physical activity and cardiorespiratory fitness. *Journal of the American Medical Association* 281, 4: 327–34.

Dunphy, Robert and Kimberly Fisher. 1994. Transportation, congestion, and density: new insights. *Transportation Research Record* 1552: 89–96.

Durkin, Maureen, Leslie Davidson, Louise Kuhn, Patricia O'Connor, and Barbara Barlow. 1994. Low-income neighborhoods and the risk of severe pediatric injury: a small-area analysis. *American Journal of Public Health* 84, 4: 587–92.

Durkin, Maureen, Danielle Laraque, Ilona Lubman, and Barbara Barlow. 1999. Epidemiology and prevention of traffic injuries to urban children and adolescents. *Pediatrics* 103, 6: E74. Available on-line at http://www.pediatrics.org/cgi/content/full/103/6/e74.

Editors of *Fortune* Magazine. 1958. *The Exploding Metropolis*. Garden City, NY: Doubleday and Company.

Ehrenhalt, Alan. 1997. The asphalt rebellion. *Governing Magazine* (October). Available on-line at http://governing.com/archive/1997/oct/roads.txt.

Ellaway, A., A. Anderson, and S. Macintyre. 1997. Does area of residence affect body size and shape? *International Journal of Obesity* 21, 4: 304–8.

Epperson, Bruce. 1994. Evaluating suitability of roadways for bicycle use: toward a cycling level-of-service standard. *Transportation Research Record* 1438: 9–16.

Eubank-Ahrens, Brenda. 1987. A Closer Look at the Users of Woonerven. In Anne Moudon (Ed.), *Public Streets for Public Use*. New York: Van Nostrand Reinhold Co., Inc.

Ewing, Reid. 2001. Impacts of traffic calming. *Transportation Quarterly* 55, 1: 33–45.

———. 1999. *Traffic Calming: State of the Practice*. Prepared for the U.S. Department of Transportation, Federal Highway Administration, Office of Safety Research and Development and Office of Human Environment; prepared by Institute of Transportation Engineers. Report number FHWA-RD-99-135.

———. 1997. *Transportation and Land Use Innovations: When You Can't Pave Your Way Out of Congestion*. Chicago: American Planning Assocation.

———. 1994. Residential street design: do the British and Australians know something Americans do not? *Transportation Research Record* 1455: 42–9.

Ewing, Reid, Padma Halidur, and G. William Page. 1994. Getting around a traditional city, a suburban planned unit development, and everything in between. *Transportation Research Record* 1466: 53–62.

Fairbanks, Robert. 1985. From better dwellings to better community: Changing approaches to the low-cost housing problem, 1890–1925. *Journal of Urban History* 11, 3: 314–34.

Fairfield, John. 1994. The scientific management of urban space: professional city planning and the legacy of progressive reform. *Journal of Urban History* 20, 2: 179–204.

Federal Highway Administration. 2001. *The Effects of Traffic Calming Measures on Pedestrian and Motorist Behavior*. Report No. FHWA-RD-00-104. McLean, VA: Turner-Fairbank Highway Research Center.

———. 1997. *Our Nation's Travel: 1995 NPTS Early Results Report*. Washington, D.C.: U.S. Department of Transportation.

———. 1994. *The National Bicycling and Walking Study. Case Study Number 1: Reasons Why Bicycling and Walking Are and Are Not Being Used More Extensively as Travel Modes*. Washington, D.C.: U.S. Department of Transportation.

Federal Interagency Forum on Aging-Related Statistics. 2000. *Older Americans*

2000: Key Indicators of Well-Being. Federal Interagency Forum on Aging-Related Statistics, Washington, DC: U.S. Government Printing Office. August 2000.

Fein, Albert. 1967. *Landscape into Cityscape: Frederick Law Olmsted's Plans for a Greater New York City.* Ithaca, NY: Cornell University Press.

Ferucci, Luigi, Brenda Penninx, Suzanne Leveille, Maria-Chiara Corti, Marco Pahor, Robert Wallace, Tamara Harris, Richard Havlik, Jack Guralnik. 2000. Characteristics of nondisabled older persons who perform poorly in objective tests of lower extremity function. *Journal of the American Geriatrics Society* 48, 9: 1102–10.

Fiscella, K. and P. Franks. 1997. Poverty or income inequality as predictor of mortality: longitudinal cohort study. *British Medical Journal* 314: 1724–7.

Fitzpatrick, Kevin and Mark LaGory. 2000. *Unhealthy Places: The Ecology of Risk in the Urban Landscape.* New York: Routledge.

Flegal, Katherine, Margaret Carroll, Cynthia Ogden, and Clifford Johnson. 2002. Prevalence and trends in obesity among U.S. adults, 1999–2000. *Journal of the American Medical Association* 288, 14: 1723–7.

Forester, John. 2001. Ideas in motion: the bicycle transportation controversy. *Transportation Quarterly* 55, 2: 7–17.

Forkenbrock, David and Lisa Schweitzer. 1997. *Environmental Justice and Transportation Investment Policy.* Iowa City, IA: Public Policy Center, University of Iowa.

Foster, Mark. 1981. *From Streetcar to Superhighway: American City Planners and Urban Transportation, 1900–1940.* Philadelphia: Temple University Press.

Frank, Lawrence. 2000. Land use and transportation interaction: implications on public health and quality of life. *Journal of Planning, Education, and Research* 20, 1: 6–22.

Frank, Lawrence, Eric Dumbaugh, and Lauren Leary. 2002. *Assessing Land Use, Transportation, Air Quality, and Health Relationships in King County, WA.* Submitted to King County (Washington) Department of Transportation. Unpublished report.

Frank, Lawrence, and Gary Pivo. 1995. Impacts of mixed use and density on utilization of three modes of travel: single-occupant vehicle, transit, and walking. *Transportation Research Record* 1466: 44–52.

Frank, Lawrence, Brian Stone Jr., and William Bachman. 2000. Linking land use with household vehicle emissions in the central Puget Sound: methodological framework and findings. *Transportation Research Part D* 5, 3: 173–96.

Freedman, D. S., L. K. Khan, W. H. Dietz, S. R. Srinivasan, and G. S. Berenson. 2001. Relationship of childhood obesity to coronary heart disease risk factors in adulthood: the Bogalusa Heart Study. *Pediatrics* 108, 3: 712–8.

Friedman, Bruce, Stephen Gordon, and John Peers. 1994. Effect of neo-traditional neighborhood design on travel characteristics. *Transportation Research Record* 1466: 63–70.

Fulton, William, Rolf Pendall, Mai Nguyen, and Alicia Harrison. 2001. *Who Sprawls Most? How Growth Patterns Differ Across the U.S.* Washington, D.C.: Brookings Institution, Center on Urban and Metropolitan Policy. Available on-line at: http://www.brook.edu/dybdocroot/es/urban/publications/fulton.pdf.

Gehl, Jan. 1987. *Life Between Buildings: Using Public Space.* New York: Van Nostrand Reinhold Co.

Gillette, Howard. 1983. The evolution of neighborhood planning: from the Progressive Era to the 1949 Housing Act. *Journal of Urban History* 9, 4: 421–44.

Go for Green/Environics. 1998. *1998 National Survey on Active Transportation: Summary Report.* Ottawa, Canada.

Grava, Sigurd. 1993. Traffic calming—can it be done in America? *Transportation Quarterly* 47, 4: 283–305.

Grunbaum, Jo Anne, Laura Kann, Steven Kinchen, Barbara Williams, James Ross, Richard Lowry, and Lloyd Kolbe. 2002. Youth risk behavior surveillance— United States, 2001. *Morbidity and Mortality Weekly Report* 51, SS04: 1–64.

Guerard, Arthur. 1903. The relation of tuberculosis to the tenement house problem. In Robert DeForest and Lawrence Veiller (Eds.), *The Tenement House Problem, Including the Report of the New York State Tenement House Commission of 1900.* Volume one (2 volumes). New York: The Macmillan Company.

Gutman, Robert. 1986. The street generation. In Stanford Anderson (Ed.), *On Streets.* Cambridge, MA: MIT Press.

Gyourko, Joseph and Witold Rybczynski. 2000. Financing New Urbanism projects: obstacles and solutions. *Housing Policy Debate* 11, 3: 733–50.

Haefeli, Ueli. 2001. *Public transport can pay. A historical analysis of transport policies in Bern (Switzerland) and Bielefeld (Germany) since 1950.* Paper presented at the 1st Swiss Transport Research Conference, Ascona, Switzerland, March 1–3, 2001.

Hall, Peter. 1996. *Cities of Tomorrow: An Intellectual History of Urban Planning and Design in the Twentieth Century.* Updated Edition. Oxford: Blackwell Publishers.

Handy, Susan. 1992. Regional versus local accessibility: neo-traditional development and its implications for non-work travel. *Built Environment* 18, 4: 253–67.

Hartman, Jan. 1993. The Delft Bicycle Network. In Rodney Tolley (Ed.), *The Greening of Urban Transport: Planning for Walking and Cycling in Western Cities.* London: Belhaven Press.

Heydecker, Wayne and Ernest Goodrich. 1929. Sunlight and daylight for urban areas. In *Neighborhood and Community Planning: Regional Survey, Volume VII.* New York: Committee on Regional Plan of New York and its Environs.

Highway Research Center. 1994. *A Compendium of Available Bicycle and Pedestrian Trip Generation Data in the United States.* Prepared for the Federal Highway Administration. Chapel Hill, N.C.: University of North Carolina.

Hillman, Mayer. 1992. *Cycling: Towards Health and Safety.* Oxford: Oxford University Press, British Medical Association.

Hillman, Mayer, John Adams, and John Whitelegg. 1990. *One False Move: A Study of Children's Independent Mobility.* London: PSI Publishing.

Holtzclaw, John. 1994. *Using Residential Patterns and Transit to Decrease Auto Dependence and Costs.* Prepared for National Resources Defense Council for California Home Energy Efficiency Rating Systems.

Howard, Ebenezer. 1946. *Garden Cities of To-morrow.* London: Faber and Faber Ltd.

Hu, Frank, Ronald Sigal, Janet Rich-Edwards, Graham Colditz, Caren Solomon, Walter Willett, Frank Speizer, and JoAnn Manson. 1999. Walking compared with vigorous physical activity and risk of type 2 diabetes in women. *Journal of the American Medical Association* 282, 15: 1433–9.

Hu, Patricia and Jennifer Young. 1999. *Summary of Travel Trends: 1995 Nationwide Personal Transportation Survey.* Prepared for U.S. Department of Transportation, Federal Highway Administration. Knoxville, TN: Oak Ridge National Laboratory.

Hubbard, Theodora. 1925. Survey of city and regional planning in the United States, 1924. *City Planning* 1, 1: 7–29.

Hubbard, Theodora and Henry Hubbard. 1929. *Our Cities Today and Tomorrow: A Survey of Planning and Zoning Progress in the United States.* Cambridge, MA: Harvard University Press.

Hülsmann, Wulf. 1993. The 'Bicycle-Friendly' Towns Project in the Federal Republic of Germany. In Rodney Tolley (ed.), *The Greening of Urban Transport: Planning for Walking and Cycling in Western Cities.* London: Belhaven Press.

Hupkes, Geurt. 1982. The law of constant travel time and trip rates. *Futures* 14, 1: 38–46.

Inam, Aseem, Jonathan Levine, and Richard Werbel. 2002. Developer-planner interaction transportation and land use sustainability. San Jose, Ca.: Mineta Transportation Institute, San Jose State University. MTI Report 01-21.

Institute of Transportation Engineers. 1999. *Traditional Neighborhood Development: Street Design Guidelines.* Washington, D.C.: Institute of Transportation Engineers.

Jackson, Kenneth. 1985. *Crabgrass Frontier: The Suburbanization of the United States.* New York: Oxford University Press.

Jacobs, Jane. 1993. *The Death and Life of Great American Cities*. New York: The Modern Library.

Jaskiewicz, Frank. 1996. *Pedestrian Level of Service Based on Trip Quality*. Philadelphia: Glatting Jackson Kercher Anglin Lopez Rinehart, Inc.

Khisty, C. Jotin. 1994. Evaluation of pedestrian facilities: Beyond the level-of-service concept. *Transportation Research Record* 1438: 45–50.

Kitamura, Ryuichi, Patricia Mokhtarian, and Laura Laidet. 1994. *A micro-analysis of land use and travel in five neighborhoods in the San Francisco Bay Area*. Davis, Calif.: Institute of Transportation Studies, University of California, Davis. Working paper number UCD-ITS-RR-94-28.

Knack, Ruth. 2002. Dense, denser, denser still. *Planning* 68, 8: 4–9.

Koplan, Jeffrey and William Dietz. 1999. Caloric imbalance and public health policy. *Journal of the American Medical Association* 282, 16: 1579–81.

Kovar, P., J. Allegrante, C. Mackenzie, M. Peterson, B. Gutin, and M. Carlson. 1992. Supervised fitness walking in patients with osteoarthritis of the knee: a randomized, controlled trial. *Annals of Internal Medicine* 116, 7: 529–34.

Krizek, Kevin. 2000. Pretest-posttest strategy for researching neighborhood-scale urban form and travel behavior. *Transportation Research Record* 1722: 48–55.

Kujala, U., Kaprio, J., Sarna, S., Koskenvuo, M. 1998. Relationship of leisure-time physical activity and mortality: the Finnish twin cohort. *Journal of the American Medical Association* 279, 6: 440–4.

Le Corbusier. 1964. *The Radiant City*. New York: Orion Press.

Leinberger, Christopher. 2001. Financing progressive development. *Capital Xchange*, May 2001. Washington, D.C.: Brookings Institution, Center on Urban and Metropolitan Policy; Boston, MA: Harvard University, Joint Center for Housing Studies. Available on-line at http://www.brook.edu/es/urban/capitalxchange/leinberger.pdf.

Leon, Arthur, J. Connett, D. Jacobs, and Rainer Rauramaa. 1987. Leisure-time physical activity levels and risk of coronary heart disease and death in the multiple risk factor intervention trial. *Journal of the American Medical Association* 258: 2388–95.

Levine, Jonathan. 1999. Access to choice. *Access* 14: 16–19. Berkeley, CA: University of California Transportation Center.

Levine, Jonathan, Aseem Inam, Richard Werbel, and Gwo-Wei Torng. 2002. *Land Use and Transportation Alternatives: Constraint or Expansion of Household Choice?* San Jose: Mineta Transportation Institute, College of Business, San Jose State University. MTI Report 01-19.

Linenger, Jerry, Charles Chesson II, and D. Stephen Nice. 1991. Physical fitness gains following simple environmental change. *American Journal of Preventative Medicine* 7, 5: 298–310.

Lipford, William and Glennon Harrison. 2000. *RS20469: Bicycle and Pedestrian Transportation Policies.* Washington, D.C.: United States Library of Congress, Congressional Research Service. Available on-line at www.cnie.org.

Logan, Thomas. 1976. The Americanization of German zoning. *Journal of the American Institute of Planners* 42, 4: 377–85.

Lubove, Roy (Ed.). 1967. *The Urban Community: Housing and Planning in the Progressive Era.* Englewood Cliffs, NJ: Prentice-Hall.

——. 1963. *Community Planning in the 1920's: The Contribution of the Regional Planning Association of America.* Pittsburgh: University of Pittsburgh Press.

——. 1962. *The Progressives and the Slums: Tenement House Reform in New York City 1890–1917.* Pittsburgh: University of Pittsburgh Press.

Malina, Robert. 2001. Tracking of physical activity across the lifespan. *President's Council on Physical Fitness and Sports Research Digest* 3, 14 (September): 1–8.

Marcuse, Peter. 1977. Housing policy and city planning: The puzzling split in the United States, 1893–1931. In Gordon Cherry (Ed.), *Shaping an Urban World.* New York: St. Martin's Press.

McGinnis, J. Michael and William Foege. 1993. Actual causes of death in the U.S. *Journal of the American Medical Association* 270, 18: 2207–12.

Melosi, Martin (Ed.). 1980. *Pollution and Reform in American Cities, 1870–1930.* Austin, TX: University of Texas Press.

Metro Regional Services. 1997. *Creating Livable Streets: Street Design Guidelines for 2040.* Portland, Ore.: Metro Regional Services, October 1997.

Moe, Ray and Kathleen Reavis. 1997. *Pedestrian Level of Service.* Fort Collins, CO: Balloffet and Associates, Inc.

Mokdad, Ali, Barbara Bowman, Earl Ford, Frank Vinicor, James Marks, and Jeffrey Koplan. 2001. The continuing epidemics of obesity and diabetes in the United States. *Journal of the American Medical Association* 286, 10: 1195–1200.

Mokdad. Ali, Mary Serdula, William Dietz, Barbara Bowman, James Marks, and Jeffrey Koplan. 1999. The spread of the obesity epidemic in the United States, 1991–1998. *Journal of the American Medical Association* 282, 16: 1519–22.

Monheim, Rolf. 1986. Pedestrianization in German towns: a process of continual development. *Built Environment* 12, 1/2: 30–43.

Moore, Robin. 1987. Streets as playgrounds. In Anne Moudon (Ed.), *Public Streets for Public Use.* New York: Van Nostrand Reinhold Co., Inc.

Morgan, W. P. 2001. Prescription of physical activity: a paradigm shift. *Quest* 53, 3: 366–82.

Moritz, W. 1998. Adult bicyclists in the United States: characteristics and riding experience in 1996. *Transportation Research Record* 1636: 1–7.

——. 1997. Survey of North American bicycle commuters: design and aggregate results. *Transportation Research Record* 1578: 91–101.

Morris, A. E. J. 1994. *History of Urban Form: Before the Industrial Revolutions.* Third Edition. Essex, England: Longman Ltd.

Morris, Jeremy and Adrianne Hardman. 1997. Walking to health. *Sports Medicine* 23, 5: 307–31.

Moudon, Anne and Richard Untermann. 1987. Grids revisited. In Anne Moudon (Ed.), *Public Streets for Public Use.* New York: Van Nostrand Reinhold Co., Inc.

Moudon, Anne, Paul Hess, Mary Snyder, Kiril Stanilov. 1997. Effects of site design on pedestrian travel in mixed-use, medium-density environments. *Transportation Research Record* 1578: 48–55.

Mumford, Lewis. 1932. The plan of New York. *The New Republic* 71, 915 (June 15, 1932): 121–6.

Murakami, Elaine and Jennifer Young. 1997. Daily travel by persons with low income. In MultiConsultant Associates, Inc., *Proceedings from the Nationwide Personal Transportation Survey Symposium.* Washington, D.C.: U.S. Department of Transportation.

Must, Aviva, Jennifer Spadano, Eugenie Coakley, Alison Field, Graham Colditz, and William Dietz. 1999. The disease burden associated with overweight and obesity. *Journal of the American Medical Association* 282, 16: 1523–9.

Myers, Dowell and Elizabeth Gearin. 2002. Current preferences and future demand for denser residential environments. *Housing Policy Debate* 12, 4: 633–57.

Myers, Renee and David Roth. 1997. Perceived benefits of and barriers to exercise and stage of exercise adoption in young adults. *Health Psychology* 16, 3: 277–83.

National Safe Kids Campaign. 2002. *Report to the Nation on Child Pedestrian Safety.* Washington, D.C.: National Safe Kids Campaign.

Nelson, Arthur and David Allen. 1997. If you build them, commuters will use them: Association between bicycle facilities and bicycle commuting. *Transportation Research Record* 1578: 79–82.

Nielson, Ole. 1993. Safe routes to school in Odense, Denmark. In Rodney Tolley (ed.), *The Greening of Urban Transport: Planning for Walking and Cycling in Western Cities.* London: Belhaven Press.

Niemeier, Deborah and G. Scott Rutherford. 1994. *1990 NPTS Report Series: Travel Mode Special Report.* Washington, D.C.: U.S. Department of Transportation, Federal Highway Administration.

Nivola, Pietro. 1999. *Laws of the Landscape: How Policies Shape Cities in Europe and America.* Washington, D.C.: Brookings Institution Press.

Oja, Pekka, Ilkka Vuori, and Olavi Paronen. 1998. Daily walking and cycling to work: their utility as health-enhancing physical activity. *Patient Education and Counseling* 33: S87–S94.

Organisation for Economic Co-operation and Development (OECD). 1998.

Safety of Vulnerable Road Users. DSTI/DOT/RTR/RS7(98)1/FINAL. Paris: OECD, Directorate for Science, Technology, and Industry, Scientific Expert Group on the Safety of Vulnerable Road Users.

Owen, Neville and Adrian Bauman. 1992. The descriptive epidemiology of a sedentary lifestyle in adult Australians. *International Journal of Epidemiology* 21, 2: 305–10.

Owens, Peter. 1993. Neighborhood form and pedestrian life: taking a closer look. *Landscape and Urban Planning* 26: 115–35.

Paffenbarger, Ralph and I-Min Lee. 1996. Physical activity and fitness for health and longevity. *Research Quarterly for Exercise and Sport* 67, Supplement to number 3: 11–28.

Painter, Kate. 1996. The influence of street lighting improvements on crime, fear and pedestrian street use after dark. *Landscape and Urban Planning* 35: 193–201.

Parsons, Brinkerhoff Quade and Douglas, Inc., Cambridge Systematics, Inc., and Calthorpe Associates. 1996. *Transit, Urban Form and the Built Environment: A Summary of Knowledge.* Transit Cooperative Research Program. Project H-1.

———. 1993a. *Building Orientation: A Supplement to The Pedestrian Environment: Volume 4B.* Portland, OR: 1000 Friends of Oregon.

———. 1993b. *The Pedestrian Environment: Volume 4A.* Portland, OR: 1000 Friends of Oregon.

Pate, Russell, Michael Pratt, Steven Blair, William Haskell, Caroline Macera, Claude Bouchard, David Buchner, Walter Ettinger, Gregory Heath, Abby King, Andrea Kriska, Arthur Leon, Bess Marcus, Jeremy Morris, Ralph Paffenbarger, Kevin Patrick, Michael Pollock, J. M. Rippe, James Sallis, Jack Wilmore. 1995. Physical activity and public health: A recommendation from the Centers for Disease Control and Prevention and the American College of Sports Medicine. *Journal of the American Medical Association* 273: 402–7.

Pedestrian Federation of America. 1995. *Walk Tall: A Citizen's Guide to Walkable Communities.* Emmaus, PA: Rodale Press, Inc.

Pendall, Rolf. 1999. Do land-use controls cause sprawl? *Environment and Planning B* 26: 555–71.

Perry, Clarence. 1939. *Housing for the Machine Age.* New York: Russell Sage Foundation.

———. 1929. The Neighborhood Unit. In *Neighborhood and Community Planning: Regional Survey, Volume VII.* New York: Committee on Regional Plan of New York and its Environs.

Pless, B., R. Verreault, L. Arsenault, J. Frappier, and J. Stulginska. 1987. The epidemiology of road accidents in children. *American Journal of Public Health* 77, 3: 358–60.

Powell, Kenneth and Steven Blair. 1994. The public health burdens of sedentary living habits: theoretical but realistic estimates. *Medicine and Science in Sports and Exercise* 26, 7: 851–6.

Powell, Kenneth, Susan Bricker, and Steven Blair. 2002. Treating inactivity. *American Journal of Preventive Medicine* 23, 2S: 1–4.

Pratt, Michael, Caroline Macera, and Guijing Wang. 2000. Higher direct medical costs associated with physical inactivity. *The Physician and Sports Medicine* 28, 10: 63–70.

Project for Public Spaces. 1993. *National Bicycling and Walking Study, FHWA Case Study No. 20: The Effects of Environmental Design on the Amount and Type of Bicycling and Walking.* Prepared for the U.S. Department of Transportation, Federal Highway Administration. Washington, D.C.

Pucher, John. 2001. Ideas in motion: cycling safety on bikeways vs. roads. *Transportation Quarterly* 55, 4: 9–11.

———. 1998. Urban transport in Germany: providing feasible alternatives to the car. *Transport Reviews* 18, 4: 285–310.

———. 1997. Bicycling boom in Germany: a revival engineered by public policy. *Transportation Quarterly* 51, 4: 31–46.

Pucher, John and Steffen Clorer. 1992. Taming the automobile in Germany. *Transportation Quarterly* 46, 3: 383–95.

Pucher, John and Lewis Dijkstra. 2000. Making walking and cycling safer: lessons from Europe. *Transportation Quarterly* 54, 3: 25–50.

Pucher, John, Charles Komanoff, and Paul Schimek. 1999. Bicycling renaissance in North America? Recent trends and alternative policies to promote bicycling. *Transportation Research Part A* 33, 7/8: 625–54.

Pucher, John and Christian Lefevre. 1996. *The Urban Transport Crisis in Europe and North America.* London: Macmillan Press Ltd.

Rapoport, Amos. 1987. Pedestrian street use: Culture and perception. In Anne Moudon (Ed.), *Public Streets for Public Use.* New York: Van Nostrand Reinhold Co., Inc.

———. 1982. *The Meaning of the Built Environment: A Nonverbal Communication Approach.* Beverly Hills, CA: Sage Publications.

Roberts, Ian, Robyn Norton, Rodney Jackson, R. Dunn, I. Hassall. 1995. Effect of environmental factors on risk of child pedestrians by motor vehicles: a case-control study. *British Medical Journal* 310: 91–4.

Rodale Press, Inc. 1995. *Pathways for People II.* Emmaus, PA: Rodale Press, Inc. Research conducted by Parkwood Research Associates, Allentown, PA. Available on-line at safety.fhwa.dot.gov/fourthlevel/pdf/pathii.pdf.

Rosen, George. 1958. *A History of Public Health.* New York: MD Publications, Inc.

Rowland, Thomas. 1999. Adolescence: a 'risk factor' for physical inactivity. *President's Council on Physical Fitness and Sports Research Digest* 3, 6 (June): 1–8.

Rowland, Thomas, and P. Freedson. 1994. Physical activity, fitness, and health in children: a closer look. *Pediatrics* 93: 669–72.

Saalman, Howard. 1971. *Haussmann: Paris Transformed.* New York: George Braziller, Inc.

Saelens, B. E., J. F. Sallis, J. Black, and D. Chen. Forthcoming. Preliminary evaluation of the Neighborhood Environment Walkability Scale and neighborhood-based differences in physical activity. Submitted to the *American Journal of Public Health.*

Saelens, Brian, Sallis, James, and Lawrence Frank. 2003. Environmental correlates of walking and cycling: findings from the transportation, urban design, and planning literatures. *Annals of Behavioral Medicine* 25: 80-91.

Sallis, James, Adrian Bauman, and Michael Pratt. 1998. Environmental and policy interventions to promote physical activity. *American Journal of Preventive Medicine* 15, 4: 379–97.

Sallis, James, William Haskell, Stephen Fortmann, Peter Wood, and Karen Vranizan. 1986. Moderate intensity physical activity and cardiovascular risk factors: the Stanford Five-City Project. *Preventative Medicine* 15: 561–8.

Sallis, James and Neville Owen. 1999. *Physical Activity and Behavioral Medicine.* Thousand Oaks, CA: Sage Publications.

———. 1990. Ecological models. In Karen Glanz, Barbara Rimer, and Frances Lewis (Eds.), *Health Behavior and Health Education: Theory, Research, and Practice.* Second Edition. New York: Jossey-Bass.

Sarkar, Sheila. 1994. Determination of service levels for pedestrians, with European examples. *Transportation Research Record* 1405: 35–42.

Schafer, Andreas and David Victor. 2000. The future mobility of the world population. *Transportation Research Part A: Policy and Practice* 34, 3: 171–205.

Schaeffer, K. H., and Elliott Sclar. 1980. *Access for All: Transportation and Urban Growth.* New York: Columbia University Press.

Schaffer, Daniel. 1982. *Garden Cities for America: The Radburn Experience.* Philadelphia: Temple University Press.

Schmid, Thomas, and Lawrence Frank. 2003. Connecting smart growth and public health: the missing links. Paper presented at the *New Partners for Smart Growth Conference,* January 30–February 1, 2003, New Orleans, Louisiana.

Schmid, Thomas, Michael Pratt, and Elizabeth Howze. 1995. Policy as intervention: environmental and policy approaches to the prevention of cardiovascular disease. *American Journal of Public Health* 85, 9: 1207–11.

Schoenborn, Charlotte, and Patricia Barnes. 2002. Leisure-time physical activity among adults: United States, 1977-98. *Advance Data from Vital and Health Sta-*

tistics, no. 325 (April 7, 2002). Hyattsville, MD: National Center for Health Statistics, Centers for Disease Control and Prevention.

Schultz, Stanley. 1989. *Constructing Urban Culture: American Cities and City Planning, 1800–1920*. Philadelphia: Temple University Press.

Schumacher, Thomas. 1986. Buildings and Streets: Notes on Configuration and Use. In Stanford Anderson (Ed.), *On Streets*. Cambridge, MA: MIT Press.

Selberg, Knut. 1996. Road and traffic environment. *Landscape and Urban Planning* 35: 153–72.

Shephard, Roy. 1997. What is the optimal type of physical activity to enhance health? *British Journal of Sports Medicine* 31, 4: 277–84.

Sies, Mary. 1987. The city transformed: nature, technology, and the suburban ideal, 1877–1917. *Journal of Urban History* 14, 1: 81–111.

Singh, N., K. Clemets, M. Fiatarone. 1997. A randomized controlled trial of progressive resistance training in depressed elders. *Journal of Gerontology* 52A: M27–M35.

Southworth, Michael. 1997. Walkable suburbs? An evaluation of neo-traditional communities at the urban edge. *Journal of the American Planning Association* 63, 1: 28–44.

Southworth, Michael, and Eran Ben-Joseph. 2003. *Streets and the Shaping of Towns and Cities*. Washington, D.C.: Island Press.

Southworth, Michael, and Eran Ben-Joseph. 1995. Street standards and the shaping of suburbia. *Journal of the American Planning Association* 61, 1: 65–81.

Southworth, Michael, and Peter Owens. 1993. The evolving metropolis: studies of community, neighborhood, and street form at the urban edge. *Journal of the American Planning Association* 59, 3: 271–87

Spann, Edward. 1996. *Designing Modern America: The Regional Planning Association of America and its Members*. Columbus, OH: Ohio State University Press.

Stamatiadis, Nikiforos. 2001. A European approach to Context Sensitive Design. *Transportation Quarterly* 55, 4: 41–8.

Stein, Clarence. *Toward New Towns for America*. 1957. New York: Reinhold Publishing Corporation.

Stephens, Mark. 2002. Children, physical activity, and public health: another call to action. *American Family Physician* 65, 6: 1033.

Stone, Neil. 1996. The clinical and economic significance of atherosclerosis. *The American Journal of Medicine* 101, 4A: 6S–9S.

Strauss, R. 1999. Childhood obesity. *Current Problems in Pediatrics* 29, 1: 5–29.

Sutton, S. B. (ed.). 1971. *Civilizing American Cities: A Selection of Frederick Law Olmsted's Writings on City Landscapes*. Boston: The Massachusetts Institute of Technology.

Szczygiel, Bonj and Robert Hewitt. 2000. Nineteenth-century medical land-scapes: John H. Rauch, Frederick Law Olmsted, and the search for salubrity. *Bulletin of the History of Medicine* 74: 708–34.

Task Force on Community Preventive Services. 2001. Increasing physical activity: a report on recommendations of the Task Force on Community Preventive Services. *Morbidity and Mortality Weekly Report* 50, RR 18: 1–16 (October 2001).

Taylor, Lloyd. 1974. *The Medical Profession and Social Reform, 1885–1945*. New York: St. Martin's Press.

Telama, R., X. Yang, L. Laakso, and J. Viikari. 1997. *American Journal of Preventive Medicine* 13, 4: 317–23.

Toll, Seymour. 1969. *Zoned American*. New York: Grossman Publishers.

Unger, Jennifer. 1995. Sedentary lifestyle as a risk factor for self-reported poor physical and mental health. *American Journal of Health Promotion* 10, 1: 15–7.

Untermann, Richard. 1987. Changing Design Standards for Streets and Roads. In Anne Moudon (Ed.), *Public Streets for Public Use*. New York: Van Nostrand Reinhold Co., Inc.

U.S. Bureau of the Census. 2001a. *Age: 2000. Census 2000 Brief*. Washington, D.C.: Census Bureau. Brief number C2kBR/01-12. Issued October 2001. Available on-line at www.census.gov/prod/2001pubs/c2kbr01-12.pdf.

———. 2001b. *Poverty in the United States: 2000*. Washington, D.C.: Census Bureau. Current Population Reports number P60-214. Issued September 2001. Available on-line at http://www.census.gov/prod/2001pubs/p60-214.pdf.

———. 2001c. *The 65 Years and Over Population: 2000. Census 2000 Brief*. Washington, D.C.: Census Bureau. Brief number C2kBR/01-10. Issued October 2001. Available on-line at http://www.census.gov/prod/2001pubs/c2kbr01-10.pdf.

U.S. Department of Health and Human Services. 1996. *Physical Activity and Health: A Report of the Surgeon General*. Centers for Disease Control and Prevention, National Center for Chronic Disease Prevention and Health Promotion.

U.S. Department of Health and Human Services, Public Health Service, Centers for Disease Control and Prevention, National Center for Chronic Disease Prevention and Health Promotion, Division of Nutrition and Physical Activity. 1999. *Promoting Physical Activity: A Guide for Community Action*. Champaign, IL: Human Kinetics.

U.S. Department of Transportation. 2001. *National Transportation Statistics 2000*. Washington, D.C.: U.S. Government Printing Office, April 2001. Publication No. BTS01-01.

U.S. Department of Transportation, Bureau of Transportation Statistics. 1999. *Pocket Guide to Transportation*. Washington, D.C.: U.S. Department of Transportation, Bureau of Transportation Statistics, December 1999. Publication No. BTS 99-06R.

Veiller, Lawrence. 1970. Housing as a Factor in Health Progress in the Past Fifty Years. In Mazyck Ravenel (Ed.), *A Half Century of Public Health*. New York: Arno Press.

———. 1929. Light. In National Conference on City Planning, *Planning Problems of Town, City and Region: Papers and Discussions at the Twenty-First National Conference on City Planning and the Problems of Congestion*. Cambridge, MA: The University Press.

———. 1916. Districting by municipal regulation. In National Conference on City Planning, *Proceedings of the Eighth National Conference on City Planning*. New York: Douglas C. McMurtrie.

———. 1911. Buildings in relation to street and site. In National Conference on City Planning, *Proceedings of the Third National Conference on City Planning*. Cambridge, MA: The University Press.

———. 1910. The safe load of population on land. In National Conference on City Planning and the Problems of Congestion, *Proceedings of the Second National Conference on City Planning and the Problems of Congestion*. Cambridge, MA: The University Press.

———. 1903. Tenement house reform in New York City, 1834–1900. In Robert DeForest and Lawrence Veiller (Eds.), *The Tenement House Problem, Including the Report of the New York State Tenement House Commission of 1900*. Volume one (2 volumes). New York: The Macmillan Company.

Volk, Laurie and Todd Zimmerman. 2001. Comment on Dowell Myers and Elizabeth Gearin's "Current preferences and future demand for denser residential environments": in praise . . . or at least acceptance . . . of ambiguity. *Housing Policy Debate* 12, 4: 675–9.

Vuchic, Vukan. 1999. *Transportation for Livable Cities*. New Brunswick, N.J.: Center for Urban Policy Research, Rutgers University.

Vuori, Ilkka, Pekka Oja, and Olavi Paronen. 1994. Physically active commuting to work: testing its potential for exercise promotion. *Medicine and Science in Sports and Exercise* 26, 7: 844–50.

Wachs, Martin. 1988. The role of transportation in the social integration of the aged. In Committee on an Aging Society, Institute of Medicine and National Research Council (Eds.), *America's Aging: The Social and Built Environment in an Older Society*. Washington, D.C.: National Academy Press

Waitzman, N. and K. Smith. 1998. Phantom of the area: poverty-area residence and mortality in the United States. *American Journal of Public Health* 88, 6: 973–6.

Waller, A., S. Barker, and A. Szocka. 1989. Childhood injury deaths: national analysis and geographic variations. *American Journal of Public Health* 79, 3: 310–15.

Wang, Guijing, Charles Helmick, Caroline Macera, Ping Zhang, and Michael Pratt. 2001. Inactivity-associated medical costs among US adults with arthritis. *Arthritis and Rheumatism* 45, 5: 439–45.

Weiss, Marc. 1987. *The Rise of the Community Builders: The American Real Estate Industry and Urban Land Planning*. New York: Columbia University Press.

Whitelegg, John. 1993. The principle of environmental traffic management. In Rodney Tolley (Ed.), *The Greening of Urban Transport: Planning for Walking and Cycling in Western Cities*. London: Belhaven Press.

Whitten, Robert. 1921. Zoning and living conditions. In National Conference on City Planning, *Proceedings of the Thirteenth Annual Conference on City Planning*. Publisher unknown.

———. 1918. The zoning of residence sections. In National Conference on City Planning, *Proceedings of the Tenth Annual Conference on City Planning*. Boston: Taylor Press.

Wigan, Marcus. 1995. Treatment of walking as a mode of transportation. *Transportation Research Record* 1487: 7–13.

Williams, Frank Backus. 1913. Restricted residence and business districts in German cities. In National Housing Association, *Housing Problems in America: Proceedings of the Third National Conference on Housing*. Cambridge, MA: The University Press.

Willis, Carol. 1993. A 3D CBD: How the 1916 Zoning Law Shaped Manhatten's Central Business District. In Todd Bressi (Ed.), *Planning and Zoning New York City*. New Brunswick, NJ: Center for Urban Policy Research, Rutgers University.

Wolfe, Charles. 1987. Streets regulating neighborhood form: A selective history. In Anne Moudon (Ed.), *Public Streets for Public Use*. New York: Van Nostrand Reinhold Co., Inc.

Wright, Frank Lloyd. 1958. *The Living City*. New York: Bramhall House.

Wright, Henry. 1913. Transit and housing. In National Housing Association, *Housing Problems in America: Proceedings of the Third National Conference on Housing*. Cambridge, MA: The University Press.

Wynne, George. 1992. *A Study of Bicycle and Pedestrian Programs in European Countries*. Prepared for the Federal Highway Administration. Washington, D.C.

Yaffe, Kristine, Deborah Barnes, Michael Nevitt, Li-Yung Lui, and Kenneth Covinsky. 2001. A prospective study of physical activity and cognitive decline in elderly women: women who walk. *Archives of Internal Medicine* 161, 14: 1703–8.

Yen, Irene and George Kaplan. 1998. Poverty area residence and changes in physical activity level: evidence from the Alameda County Study. *American Journal of Public Health* 88, 11: 1709–12.

Zein, Sany, Erica Geddes, Suzanne Hemsing, and Mavis Johnson. 1997. Safety benefits of traffic calming. *Transportation Research Record* 1578: 3–10.

Lawrence Frank is the Bombardier Chair of Sustainable Urban Transportation Systems in the School of Community and Regional Planning at the University of British Columbia and formerly an associate professor of City and Regional Planning at Georgia Tech. He specializes in researching the relationships between urban form, travel choice, air quality, and public health. He is a registered landscape architect.

Peter Engelke is a research associate in the Georgia Tech Research Institute in Atlanta, Georgia, where his research has focused on the relationships between urban form and public health. He also has research interests in the areas of urban and environmental history and in sustainable development. He holds graduate degrees in political science from Indiana University and in public policy from the University of Maryland.

Thomas Schmid received his doctorate from West Virginia University in Behavioral Psychology and completed a Post Doctoral Fellowship in Epidemiology at the University of Minnesota. Dr. Schmid is coordinator of the Active Community Environments (ACES) team at the Centers for Disease Control and Prevention (CDC), Nutrition and Physical Activity Branch. Dr. Schmid provides technical assistance on the design, application, and evaluation of interventions designed to improve health. At the national level these efforts focus on state and local health departments, academic research centers, and other federal agencies. International assistance is provided through the World Health Organization, the World Bank, and the Ministries of Health in Russia and various countries in East Africa and Latin America.

ISLAND PRESS BOARD OF DIRECTORS

Victor M. Sher, Esq., *Chair*
Environmental Lawyer, Sher & Leff

Dane A. Nichols, *Vice-Chair*
Environmentalist

Carolyn Peachey, *Secretary*
President
Campbell, Peachey & Associates

Drummond Pike, *Treasurer*
President, The Tides Foundation

Robert E . Baensch
Director, Center for Publishing
New York University

David C. Cole
President, Aquaterra, Inc.

Catherine M. Conover
Chair, Board of Directors
Quercus LLC

Henry Reath
President, Collectors Reprints Inc.

Will Rogers
President, Trust for Public Land

Charles C. Savitt
President, Center for Resource Economics/
Island Press

Susan E. Sechler
Senior Advisor on Biotechnology Policy
The Rockefeller Foundation

Peter R. Stein
General Partner
The Lyme Timber Company

Diana Wall, Ph.D.
Director and Professor
Natural Resource Ecology Laboratory
Colorado State University

Wren Wirth
President, The Winslow Foundation

ABOUT ISLAND PRESS

Island Press is the only nonprofit organization in the United States whose principal purpose is the publication of books on environmental issues and natural resource management. We provide solutions-oriented information to professionals, public officials, business and community leaders, and concerned citizens who are shaping responses to environmental problems.

In 2003, Island Press celebrates its nineteenth anniversary as the leading provider of timely and practical books that take a multidisciplinary approach to critical environmental concerns. Our growing list of titles reflects our commitment to bringing the best of an expanding body of literature to the environmental community throughout North America and the world.

Support for Island Press is provided by The Nathan Cummings Foundation, Geraldine R. Dodge Foundation, Doris Duke Charitable Foundation, Educational Foundation of America, The Charles Engelhard Foundation, The Ford Foundation, The George Gund Foundation, The Vira I. Heinz Endowment, The William and Flora Hewlett Foundation, Henry Luce Foundation, The John D. and Catherine T. MacArthur Foundation, The Andrew W. Mellon Foundation, The Moriah Fund, The Curtis and Edith Munson Foundation, National Fish and Wildlife Foundation, The New-Land Foundation, Oak Foundation, The Overbrook Foundation, The David and Lucile Packard Foundation, The Pew Charitable Trusts, The Rockefeller Foundation, The Winslow Foundation, and other generous donors.

The opinions expressed in this book are those of the author(s) and do not necessarily reflect the views of these foundations.